COLOR ATLAS & SYNOPSIS OF
Clinical Ophthalmology

Pediatric
Ophthalmology

SECOND EDITION

EDITOR
Leonard B. Nelson, MD, MBA
Director, Strabismus Center
Co-Director, Pediatric Ophthalmology and Ocular Genetics
Wills Eye Hospital
Associate Professor of Ophthalmology and Pediatrics
Jefferson Medical College of Thomas Jefferson University
Philadelphia, Pennsylvania

SECTION EDITORS
Michael J. Bartiss, OD, MD
Caroline DeBenedictis, MD
Kammi B. Gunton, MD
Judith B. Lavrich, MD
Kara C. LaMattina, MD
Alex V. Levin, MD, MHSc, FRCSC
Scott E. Olitsky, MD
Bruce M. Schnall, MD
Aldo Vagge, MD, PhD student
Barry N. Wasserman, MD

SERIES EDITOR
Christopher J. Rapuano, MD
Director and Attending Surgeon, Cornea Service
Co-Director, Refractive Surgery Department
Wills Eye Hospital
Professor of Ophthalmology
Sidney Kimmel Medical College at Thomas Jefferson University
Philadelphia, Pennsylvania

Wills Eye Hospital

COLOR ATLAS & SYNOPSIS OF
Clinical Ophthalmology

Pediatric
Ophthalmology

SECOND EDITION

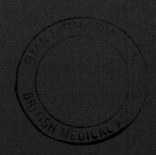

Wolters Kluwer

Philadelphia • Baltimore • New York • London
Buenos Aires • Hong Kong • Sydney • Tokyo

Acquisitions Editor: Chris Teja
Editorial Coordinator: Lauren Pecarich
Marketing Manager: Rachel Mante Lueng
Production Project Manager: David Saltzberg
Design Coordinator: Stephen Druding
Manufacturing Coordinator: Beth Welsh
Prepress Vendor: S4Carlisle Publishing Services

Second Edition

9 8 7 6 5 4 3 2 1

Printed in China

Library of Congress Cataloging-in-Publication Data

ISBN-13: 978-1-4963-6304-6
ISBN-10: 1-4963-6304-3

Cataloging-in-Publication data available on request from the Publisher.

LWW.com

To my wife, Helene, for her understanding, patience, and support.
To my children, Jen, Kim, and Brad, who have taught me what is important in life.
To my sons-in-law, Josh and Justin, and daughter-in-law, Julie, who all embody the meaning of family.
To my grandsons, Jake, Ryan, Brandon, Joey, and Jordan,
and granddaughters, Lily and Chloe, who never cease to amaze me.

And to the memory of several individuals who passed away recently and
who had a profound effect on my personal and professional life:
Dean Henry S. Coleman, whose extraordinary guidance through
my college years at Columbia University fine-tuned my future goals.
A. Stone Freedberg, MD, who was instrumental in my matriculating and
succeeding as a medical student at Harvard Medical School.
Marshall M. Parks, MD, who taught me pediatric ophthalmology and
whose skills in all aspects of the subspecialty I have always tried to emulate.

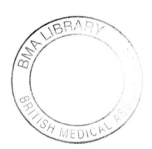
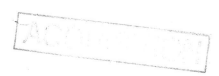

Editors

SERIES EDITOR

Christopher J. Rapuano, MD
Director and Attending Surgeon
Cornea Service
Co-Director
Refractive Surgery Department
Wills Eye Hospital
Professor of Ophthalmology
Sidney Kimmel Medical College at
    Thomas Jefferson University
Philadelphia, Pennsylvania

EDITOR

Leonard B. Nelson, MD, MBA
Director, Strabismus Center
Co-Director, Pediatric Ophthalmology and
    Ocular Genetics
Wills Eye Hospital
Associate Professor of Ophthalmology
    and Pediatrics
Jefferson Medical College of Thomas
    Jefferson University
Philadelphia, Pennsylvania

SECTION EDITORS

Michael J. Bartiss, OD, MD
Private Practice
Family Eye Care of the Carolinas
Aberdeen, North Carolina
Director of NICU Eye Services
FirstHealth of the Carolinas
Pinehurst, North Carolina

Caroline DeBenedictis, MD
Attending
Department of Pediatric Ophthalmology
Wills Eye Hospital
Clinical Instructor
Department of Ophthalmology
Thomas Jefferson University Hospital
Philadelphia, Pennsylvania

Kammi B. Gunton, MD
Assistant Professor
Department of Pediatric Ophthalmology
Wills Eye Hospital
Associate Professor
Department of Ophthalmology
Sidney Kimmel Medical College at Thomas
    Jefferson University
Philadelphia, Pennsylvania

Kara C. LaMattina, MD
Assistant Professor
Department of Ophthalmology
Boston University School of Medicine
Boston Medical Centre
Boston, Massachusetts

Judith B. Lavrich, MD
Associate Surgeon
Department of Pediatric Ophthalmology and
    Ocular Genetics
Wills Eye Hospital
Clinical Instructor
Sidney Kimmel Medical College at Thomas
    Jefferson University
Philadelphia, Pennsylvania

Alex V. Levin, MD, MHSc, FRCSC
Chief
Pediatric Ophthalmology and Ocular Genetics
Wills Eye Hospital
Professor
Ophthalmology and Pediatrics
Sidney Kimmel Medical College at Thomas
    Jefferson University
Philadelphia, Pennsylvania

Scott E. Olitsky, MD
Professor
Department of Ophthalmology
University of Missouri—Kansas City School of
    Medicine
Chief
Section of Ophthalmology
Children's Mercy Hospitals and Clinics
Kansas City, Missouri

Bruce M. Schnall, MD
Associate Surgeon
Department of Pediatric Ophthalmology
Wills Eye Hospital
Philadelphia, Pennsylvania

Aldo Vagge, MD, PhD Student
Attending Physician
Faculty Member
University Eye Clinic–Pediatric Ophthalmology
and Strabismus Service
Department of Neuroscience, Rehabilitation,
Ophthalmology, Genetics, Maternal and Child
Health (DiNOGMI)
University of Genoa
IRCCS Policlinic Hospital San Martino
Genoa, Italy

Barry N. Wasserman, MD
Associate Professor
Department of Ophthalmology
Sidney Kimmel Medical College at Thomas
Jefferson University
Clinical Instructor
Department of Pediatric Ophthalmology,
Strabismus and Ocular Genetics
Wills Eye Hospital
Philadelphia, Pennsylvania

Contributors

Alok S. Bansal, MD
Fellow
Vitreoretinal Surgery
Retina Service
Wills Eye Hospital
Philadelphia, Pennsylvania
UCSF VA Medical Center
San Francisco, California

Michael J. Bartiss, OD, MD
Private Practice
Family Eye Care of the Carolinas
Aberdeen, North Carolina
Director of NICU Eye Services
FirstHealth of the Carolinas
Pinehurst, North Carolina

Caroline DeBenedictis, MD
Attending
Department of Pediatric Ophthalmology
Wills Eye Hospital
Clinical Instructor
Department of Ophthalmology
Thomas Jefferson University Hospital
Philadelphia, Pennsylvania

Anuradha Ganesh, MD
Fellow
Pediatric Ophthalmology and
    Ocular Genetics
Wills Eye Hospital
Philadelphia, Pennsylvania
Department of Ophthalmology
Sultan Qaboos University Hospital
Sultanate of Oman

Debra A. Goldstein, MD
Magerstadt Professor of
    Ophthalmology
Department of Ophthalmology
Northwestern University Feinberg School
    of Medicine
Director, Uveitis Service
Department of Ophthalmology
Northwestern Memorial Hospital
Chicago, Illinois

Kammi B. Gunton, MD
Assistant Professor
Department of Pediatric Ophthalmology
Wills Eye Hospital
Associate Professor
Department of Ophthalmology
Sidney Kimmel Medical College at Thomas
    Jefferson University
Philadelphia, Pennsylvania

Kara C. LaMattina, MD
Assistant Professor
Department of Ophthalmology
Boston University School of Medicine
Boston Medical Centre
Boston, Massachusetts

Judith B. Lavrich, MD
Associate Surgeon
Department of Pediatric Ophthalmology and
    Ocular Genetics
Wills Eye Hospital
Clinical Instructor
Department of Ophthalmology
Sidney Kimmel Medical College at Thomas
    Jefferson University
Philadelphia, Pennsylvania

Alex V. Levin, MD, MHSc, FRCSC
Chief
Pediatric Ophthalmology and Ocular Genetics
Wills Eye Hospital
Professor
Ophthalmology and Pediatrics
Sidney Kimmel Medical College at Thomas
    Jefferson University
Philadelphia, Pennsylvania

Leonard B. Nelson, MD, MBA
Director, Strabismus Center
Co-Director, Pediatric Ophthalmology and
    Ocular Genetics
Wills Eye Hospital
Associate Professor of Ophthalmology and Pediatrics
Jefferson Medical College of Thomas Jefferson
    University
Philadelphia, Pennsylvania

Scott E. Olitsky, MD
Professor
Department of Ophthalmology
University of Missouri—Kansas City School
   of Medicine
Chief
Section of Ophthalmology
Children's Mercy Hospitals and Clinics
Kansas City, Missouri

Bruce M. Schnall, MD
Associate Surgeon
Department of Pediatric Ophthalmology
Wills Eye Hospital
Philadelphia, Pennsylvania

Emily Schnall, BFA
Independent freelance artist

Carol L. Shields, MD
Professor of Ophthalmology
Thomas Jefferson University Hospital
Co-Director
Oncology Service
Wills Eye Hospital
Philadelphia, Pennsylvania

Anya A. Trumler, MD
Fellow in Pediatric Ophthalmology and
   Ocular Genetics
Wills Eye Hospital
Philadelphia, Pennsylvania

Aldo Vagge, MD, PhD Student
Attending Physician
Faculty Member
University Eye Clinic–Pediatric Ophthalmology
   and Strabismus Service
Department of Neuroscience, Rehabilitation,
   Ophthalmology, Genetics, Maternal and Child
   Health (DiNOGMI)
University of Genoa
IRCCS Policlinic Hospital San Martino
Genoa, Italy

Barry N. Wasserman, MD
Associate Professor
Department of Ophthalmology
Sidney Kimmel Medical College at Thomas
   Jefferson University
Clinical Instructor
Department of Pediatric Ophthalmology,
   Strabismus and Ocular Genetics
Wills Eye Hospital
Philadelphia, Pennsylvania

About the Series

The beauty of the atlas/synopsis concept is the powerful combination of illustrative photographs and a summary approach to the text. Ophthalmology is a very visual discipline that lends itself wonderfully to clinical photographs. Whereas the seven ophthalmic subspecialties in this series—Cornea, Retina, Glaucoma, Oculoplastics, Neuro-ophthalmology, Uveitis, and Pediatrics—employ varying levels of visual recognition, a relatively standard format for the text is used for all volumes.

The goal of the series is to provide an up-to-date clinical overview of the major areas of ophthalmology for students, residents, and practitioners in all the health care professions. The abundance of large, excellent-quality photographs (both in print and online) and concise, outline-form text will help achieve that objective.

Christopher J. Rapuano
Series Editor

Preface

Wills Eye Hospital has been my "academic home" for over 30 years. During that time, I have witnessed remarkable changes in pediatric ophthalmology as it has become a more established and rapidly expanding subspecialty. Although many changes have occurred at Wills over those years, certain things have remained constant, including the outstanding faculty, fellows, residents, and staff, as well as the commitment to excellent patient care and academic endeavors. Wills is a rich storehouse of clinical material and has provided the major background for this book. In particular, the Pediatric Ophthalmology and Ocular Genetics Department at Wills, which cares for thousands of children each year, provides a rare opportunity for the study of an extremely wide variety of pediatric ocular disorders. It has been a pleasure to oversee the production of this book because each contributor has been part of the "Wills family."

The advances that have occurred in the understanding of pediatric ocular disease and newer modalities of treatment require a constant updating of knowledge about these conditions. This text was written in an effort to provide practicing ophthalmologists, pediatric ophthalmologists, and residents in training with a concise update of the clinical findings and the most recent treatment available for a wide spectrum of childhood ocular diseases. The disorders are grouped according to the specific ocular structure involved. The atlas format should provide readers with a clear and succinct outline of the disease entities and stimulate a more detailed pursuit of the specific ocular disorders.

Leonard B. Nelson
Editor

Acknowledgments

It is with pleasure and gratitude that I acknowledge a number of individuals who helped make this publication possible. I appreciate the members of the Audio-Visual Department at Wills Eye Hospital, Roger Barone and Jack Scully, who helped in the preparation of many of the photographs. I am grateful to Katurrah Hayman for her exceptional secretarial skills. I am indebted to Louise Biekig, the developmental editor, for her continuous suggestions and help throughout the preparation of this book. Finally, I wish to thank all the authors who gave of their time, unselfishly, in the writing of this book.

Contents

Wills Eye Hospital

COLOR ATLAS & SYNOPSIS OF
Clinical Ophthalmology

Pediatric
Ophthalmology

SECOND EDITION

Abnormalities Affecting the Eye as a Whole

Judith B. Lavrich ∎

ANOPHTHALMIA

Anophthalmia, also known as anophthalmos, is a congenital anomaly that is characterized by the complete absence of ocular tissue within the orbit. **Primary** or **true anophthalmia** is a very rare condition and can involve one or both eyes. Extreme microphthalmos is far more common and can be mistaken for this condition. Anophthalmia has a prevalence of 0.18 per 10,000 births and has no racial or sexual predilection.

Etiology

During embryogenesis, there is an arrest in the development of the neuroectoderm of the primary optic vesicle, which stems from the anterior neural plate of the neural tube.

Anophthalmia is most frequently idiopathic and sporadic but can be inherited as a dominant, recessive, or sex-linked trait. It is associated with maternal infections during pregnancy (e.g., toxoplasmosis, rubella) as well as syndromes with craniofacial malformations (e.g., Goldenhar, Hallermann-Streiff, Waardenburg syndromes). It is linked with genetic defects, including trisomies 13 to 15; chromosomal deletion in band 14q22-23 with associated polydactyly; and mutations involving *SOX2*, *RBP4*, and *OTX2*.

Signs

- The eye is the stimulus for proper growth of the orbital region; therefore, an infant born with anophthalmia has the following:
  - Orbital findings
  - Small orbital rim and entrance
  - Reduced size of bony orbital cavity
  - Globe is completely absent.
  - Extraocular muscles are usually absent.
  - Lacrimal gland and ducts may be absent.
  - Small or maldeveloped optic foramen
- Eyelid findings
  - Narrow palpebral fissures
  - Foreshortening of the eyelids
  - Shrunken conjunctival fornices
  - Levator function is decreased or absent with poor eyelid folds.
  - Contracture of the orbicularis oculi muscle

Symptoms

- Unilateral or bilateral blindness because of the absence of the globe(s)

Differential Diagnosis

- Microphthalmos, which includes the following:
  - Secondary anophthalmos: the development of the eye begins but gets arrested, resulting in only residual eye tissue or extreme microphthalmos.
  - Degenerative anophthalmos: there is formation of the optic vesicle, but subsequent degeneration occurs because of lack of blood supply or other causes.
- Cryptophthalmos: abnormal fusion of the entire eyelid margin with absence of the eyelashes
- Cystic eye: a cyst of neuroglial tissue lacking normal ocular structures

Diagnostic Evaluation

- Anomalous eyelid and orbital features (Fig. 1-1)
- Ultrasound imaging: B-scan ultrasonography of the orbit will show a complete absence of the globe. After 22 weeks' gestation, transvaginal ultrasonography can detect eye malformations, but its sensitivity in the detection of anophthalmia is not known.
- Magnetic resonance imaging (MRI) of the head and orbits: MRI will show the soft tissue within the orbital cavity (Fig. 1-2). Associated intracranial abnormalities can also be evaluated. Individuals with bilateral anophthalmos may have a related hypoplastic or absent optic chiasm as well as agenesis or dysgenesis of the corpus callosum.
- Computed tomography (CT) scan of the head and orbits: CT scan will image the bony changes and intracranial and craniofacial abnormalities seen with anophthalmia.

Treatment

- Medical care
  - Orbital conformers can be placed in the orbital cavity to stimulate growth of the bony orbit (Fig. 1-3). As the orbit grows, the conformers are changed and progressively increased in size to further expand the orbital cavity. This serial augmentation takes time and cooperation from both the patient and the parents.
  - Contraction and reversal of the benefit often occur if the conformer is left out of the orbit for a significant amount of time. With unilateral anophthalmos, the family should be aware that, most likely, the final result will not mirror the normal healthy orbit.
  - An ocular prosthesis can be fitted over the conformer to simulate the eye and improve appearance.
- Surgical care
  - The small bony cavity is a cosmetic deformity that may not allow proper fitting of a prosthesis. Therefore, surgery may be indicated for either of these problems.
  - Inflatable tissue expanders are used if conformers are not well tolerated or cannot be fit. The inflatable silicone expander is surgically positioned deep in the orbit and is accessed through a tube placed at the lateral orbital rim. The expander is filled with saline and gradually reinflated on a weekly or biweekly schedule. Compared with solid conformers, inflatable expanders may allow more rapid and extensive expansion of the bony orbit. When the desired volume is achieved, the port and bladder need to be removed and replaced with a permanent implant.
  - Hydrogel (methyl methacrylate and N-vinylpyrrolidone) expanders are self-expanding hydrophilic expanders that are implanted in the orbital tissue in their dry, contracted state through a small

incision. The implant gradually expands in size by osmotic absorption of surrounding tissue fluid. The benefit of this method is the controlled self-expansion, reducing the risk of tissue atrophy, and without the need for repeat fittings or surgery.

■ Dermal fat grafting, which involves bio-compatible grafts that grow slowly over time, can be a good option to restore volume to the hypoplastic orbit. The graft is harvested from a second surgical site, typically the buttocks. However, the graft compatibility and growth can be variable. In some cases, the fat can atrophy. Rarely, the fat can hypertrophy, necessitating debulking.

■ Injectable calcium hydroxylapatite (Radiesse) is a semipermanent dermal filler that has been reported as a new, simple, cost-effective technique to treat volume deficiency in the anophthalmic orbit in adults. Augmentation is accomplished with serial injections of the filler until adequate volumization is achieved. The results have shown lasting effect in the orbit of 1 year or more.

■ Orbitocranial advancement surgery is used for orbital expansion if conformers and expanders are unsuccessful. This method involves multiple osteotomies to divide the periocular bones and advancing them forward and outward with bone grafts and plates.

■ Because the foreshortening of the eyelids may limit the passage of a large conformer, a lateral canthotomy or cantholysis may be needed to increase the horizontal length of the palpebral fissure. Other methods to lengthen the eyelids may include skin, mucosal, or cartilage grafts.

Prognosis

● Severe cosmetic deformities can result from anophthalmia, especially if not treated early. Even with proper treatment, the results are often cosmetically suboptimal, with incomplete expansion of the orbit, malformations and immobility of the eyelids, and complete immobility of the ocular prosthesis.

● Psychosocial issues caused by absence of an eye and facial disfigurement can result. Referral for psychological counseling may be indicated for these children.

REFERENCES

Bardakiian T, Weiss A, Schneider AS. Anophthalmia/microphthalmia overview. In: Pagon RA, Bird TC, Dolan CR, Stephens K, eds. *GeneReviews*. Seattle, WA: University of Washington; 2007:1993–2004.

Bernardino R. Congenital anophthalmia: a review of dealing with volume. *Middle East Afr J Ophthalmol.* 2010;17:156–160.

https://en.wikipedia.org/wiki/Anophthalmia

Verma AS, Fitzpatrick DR. Anophthalmia and microphthalmia. *Orphanet J Rare Dis.* 2007;2:47.

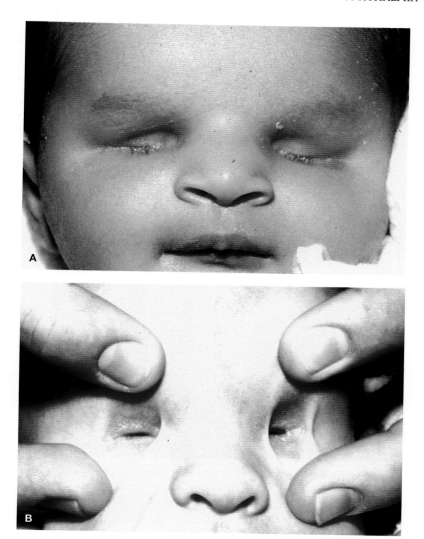

FIGURE 1-1. Anophthalmia. A. External examination of bilateral anophthalmia. **B.** Clinical examination of bilateral anophthalmia showing empty orbits. (Courtesy of Leonard B. Nelson, MD.)

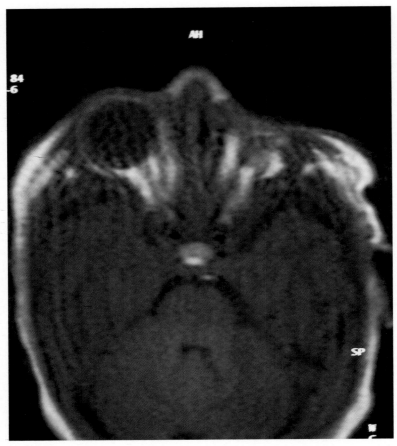

FIGURE 1-2. Anophthalmia. Magnetic resonance image showing unilateral anophthalmia with absence of the globe. (Courtesy of Carol Shields, MD.)

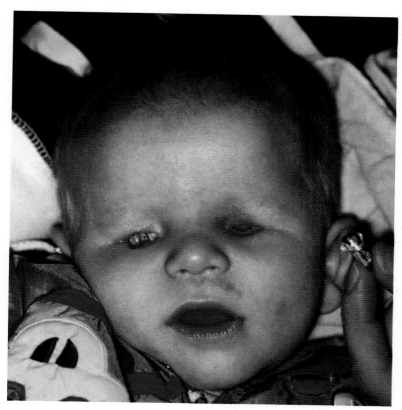

FIGURE 1-3. Anophthalmia. Fitting orbital conformers in bilateral "clinical anophthalmia" (severe microphthalmia). (Courtesy of Bruce Schnall, MD.)

MICROPHTHALMIA

Microphthalmia is a congenital unilateral or bilateral condition in which the globe has a reduced axial length that is at least two standard deviations below the mean for age. The appearance of the globe and the severity of axial length reduction define the classification of microphthalmia:

● Simple or pure microphthalmia: an eye that is anatomically intact except for its short axial length. Simple microphthalmia is suspected in the presence of high hyperopia (≥8 diopters) or microcornea. Visual loss can occur in a subset of microphthalmos associated with posterior segment abnormalities.

● Severe microphthalmia: an eye that is severely reduced in size, with an axial length of less than 10 mm at birth or less than 12 mm after age 1 year and a corneal diameter of less than 4 mm (**Fig. 1-4**). The globe may be inconspicuous on clinical examination, but remnants of ocular tissue, an optic nerve, and extraocular muscles will be seen with imaging.

● Complex microphthalmia: a globe with reduced size associated with developmental ocular malformations of the anterior or posterior segment (or both).

There are two types of microphthalmos: noncolobomatous and colobomatous (microphthalmos with cyst) (**Fig. 1-5**). The prevalence of microphthalmia is 1.5 per 10,000 births. There is no racial or sexual predilection.

Etiology

Microphthalmia results from an arrest in the development at any stage during the growth of the optic vesicle.

● Environmental: prenatal exposure of alcohol, thalidomide, retinoic acid, or rubella

● Heritable: via autosomal dominant, recessive, or X-linked inheritance

   ■ Multiple chromosomal abnormalities

   ■ Single-gene disorders causing syndromic microphthalmia (e.g., CHARGE [coloboma of the eye or central nervous system anomalies, heart defects, atresia of the choanae, retardation of growth or development, genital or urinary defects, and ear anomalies or deafness]; Lenz microphthalmia; Goltz, Aicardi, Walker-Warburg, and Meckel-Gruber syndromes, Norrie disease; incontinentia pigmenti)

   ■ Other genes: *SIX6, SHH, VSX2, RAX* and others.

● Unknown causes: Goldenhar syndrome; cases associated with basal encephalocele and other central nervous system anomalies

Signs

● Significant variability exists, depending on the severity of the microphthalmos.

   ■ Orbital findings

      ▶ Small orbital rim and entrance

      ▶ Reduced size of bony orbital cavity

      ▶ Globe is extremely small and can be malformed.

      ▶ Extraocular muscles are present but are usually hypoplastic.

      ▶ Lacrimal gland and ducts are present but are usually hypoplastic.

      ▶ Optic nerve is present but is usually hypoplastic.

      ▶ Small or maldeveloped optic foramen

   ■ Eyelid findings

      ▶ Narrow palpebral fissures

      ▶ Foreshortening of the eyelids

      ▶ Shrunken conjunctival fornices

      ▶ Levator function is decreased or absent with poor eyelid folds.

      ▶ Contracture of the orbicularis oculi muscle

Symptoms

● The extent of visual loss depends on the severity of the microphthalmos and the presence of related anomalies.

Differential Diagnosis

● Microcornea with a normal-sized globe

● High hyperopia

Diagnostic Evaluation

● Anomalous eyelid and orbital features

● Clinical examination looking for evidence of a cornea or globe

◾ Palpation of the orbit to estimate globe size

◾ Measurement of corneal diameter (normal range, 9.0–10.5 mm in neonates)

● B-scan ultrasonography to evaluate the internal structures of the globe (**Fig. 1-6A**)

● CT scan or MRI of the brain and orbits to evaluate the size of the globe and its internal structures, the presence of optic nerve and extraocular muscles, and brain anatomy (**Fig. 1-6B and C**)

Treatment

● For severe microphthalmia, the treatment is the same as for anophthalmia.

● For simple or complex microphthalmos with vision

◾ Treatment of amblyopia: patching of the healthy eye to stimulate as much potential vision as possible

◾ Protection of the healthy eye in children with unilateral involvement

◾ Visual aids and other visual resources for children with reduced vision

◾ Orbital conformers: placed over the microphthalmic eye to stimulate growth of the bony orbit. These can be painted or with the pupil left clear for vision.

◾ Ocular prosthesis: can be fitted over the globe to improve appearance, if needed

Prognosis

● For severe microphthalmia, the prognosis is the same as for anophthalmia.

● For simple microphthalmia, the visual prognosis depends on the severity of the condition and the associated ocular abnormalities.

REFERENCES

Bardakiian T, Weiss A, Schneider AS. Anophthalmia/microphthalmia overview. In: Pagon RA, Bird TC, Dolan CR, Stephens K, eds. *GeneReviews*. Seattle, WA: University of Washington; 2007:1993–2004.

Bernardino R. Congenital anophthalmia: a review of dealing with volume. *Middle East Afr J Ophthalmol.* 2010;17:156–160.

https://en.wikipedia.org/wiki/Microphthalmia

Verma AS, Fitzpatrick DR. Anophthalmia and microphthalmia. *Orphanet J Rare Dis.* 2007;2:47.

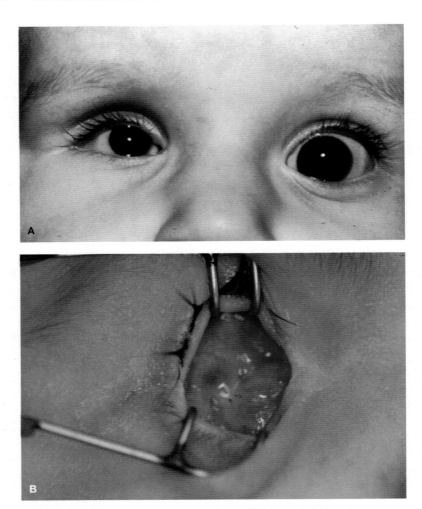

FIGURE 1-4. Microphthalmia. **A.** Unilateral microphthalmia. **B.** Severe microphthalmia.

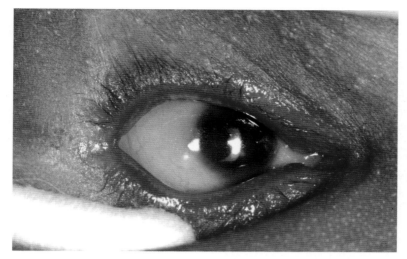

FIGURE 1-5. **Microphthalmia.** Microphthalmia with a cyst. (Courtesy of Carol Shields, MD.)

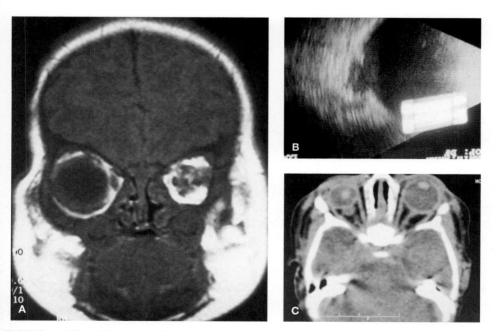

FIGURE 1-6. **Microphthalmia. A.** Magnetic resonance image showing unilateral microphthalmia. Note the presence of extraocular muscles and an optic nerve. **B.** B-scan ultrasonography of microphthalmia with a cyst showing a posterior staphyloma. **C.** Computed tomography scan of microphthalmia with a cyst showing disorganization of ocular tissues and posterior cyst. (Courtesy of Carol Shields, MD.)

NANOPHTHALMIA

Nanophthalmia is a subtype of simple microphthalmia. It is a congenital and typically bilateral condition (Fig. 1-7), although it can be unilateral. It is characterized by reduced globe volume, although the eye is otherwise grossly normal.

Etiology

- Nanophthalmia results from an arrest in the growth of the eye during the embryonic stage and may result from a smaller optic vesicle anlage.
- Most cases are sporadic, but both autosomal recessive and autosomal dominant inheritance have been reported.

Signs

- Reduced axial length of the globe (<20 mm)
- Very high hyperopia (>10 diopters)
- Reduced corneal diameter
- Lens is normal in size.
- Shallow anterior chamber
- Thick sclera
- Fundus may show crowded optic disc, vascular tortuosity, and macular hypoplasia.
- Because of the anatomy, these eyes have a high risk for angle-closure glaucoma. They tolerate intraocular surgery poorly with a high rate of complications, including uveal effusion and retinal detachment.

Differential Diagnosis

- High hyperopia in a normal eye

Diagnostic Evaluation

- Measurement of corneal diameter
- A-scan to measure the axial length of the eye
- Pentacam and ultrasound biomicroscopy to image the anterior chamber and assess its depth (Fig. 1-8).

Treatment

- Management of narrow-angle or angle-closure glaucoma is initially medical, although the response to treatment is typically poor, and miotics may even worsen the condition by relaxing the lens zonules. Peripheral laser iridotomy may be moderately successful. Caution must be used with fistulizing glaucoma surgery because postoperative malignant glaucoma can ensue. Laser trabeculoplasty, if performed, must be done early before permanent damage to the outflow mechanism occurs.
- Removal of the lens must be anticipated and can be complicated by uveal effusion and nonrhegmatogenous retinal detachments. Although challenging in these high-risk eyes, small-incision cataract surgery is safe and diminishes the need for prophylactic sclerotomies.

Prognosis

- The prognosis for vision is good if glaucoma is treated early and successfully.

REFERENCES

Bardakiian T, Weiss A, Schneider AS. Anophthalmia/microphthalmia overview. In: Pagon RA, Bird TC, Dolan CR, Stephens K, eds. *GeneReviews*. Seattle,WA: University of Washington; 2007:1993–2004.

Bernardino R. Congenital anophthalmia: a review of dealing with volume. *Middle East Afr J Ophthalmol.* 2010;17:156–160.

https://eyewiki.aao.org/Nanophthalmos

Sharan S, Grigg JR, Higgins RA. Nanophthalmos: ultrasound biomicroscopy and Pentacam assessment of angle structures before and after cataract surgery. *J Cataract Refract Surg.* 2006;32:1052–1055.

Verma AS, Fitzpatrick DR. Anophthalmia and microphthalmia. *Orphanet J Rare Dis.* 2007;2:47.

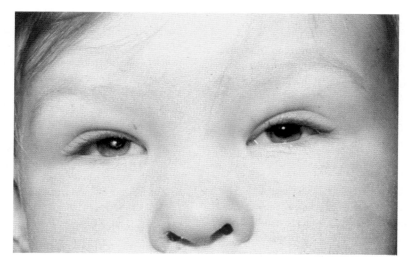

FIGURE 1-7. Bilateral nanophthalmia. Note the reduced corneal diameter.

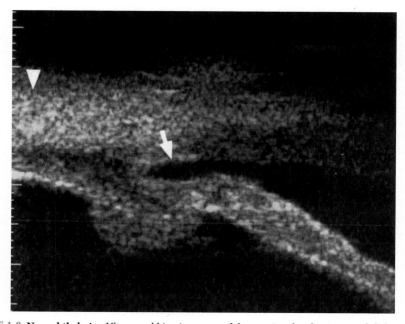

FIGURE 1-8. Nanophthalmia. Ultrasound biomicroscopy of the anterior chamber in nanophthalmos. The iris is bowed forward, creating a plateau-like configuration of the narrow angle (*arrow*), and the anterior sclera (*arrowhead*) shows increased thickness. (From Buys YM, Pavlin CJ. Retinitis pigmentosa, nanophthalmos, and optic disc drusen: a case report. *Ophthalmology.* 1999;106:619–622.)

TYPICAL COLOBOMA

The term *coloboma* is derived from the Greek *koloboma*, meaning mutilated or curtailed. It is a congenital malformation and refers to a notch, gap, hole, or fissure in any of the ocular structures. Typical colobomas are frequently bilateral and are often associated with microphthalmia.

Etiology

● "Typical" colobomata are caused by defective closure of the optic fissure during the fifth to seventh weeks of fetal life and because of the location of the fetal fissure and are found in the inferonasal quadrant in the eye. ("Atypical" colobomata are less frequent malformations located outside the inferotemporal quadrant, for which the etiology is still unclear.)

● Most cases are idiopathic and sporadic, but all types of inheritance (i.e., autosomal dominant, autosomal recessive, and X-linked) have been reported and may be associated with various syndromes, such as CHARGE, Meckel-Gruber, Lenz microphthalmia, Aicardi, Patau, and Edwards syndromes. The prevalence of coloboma is 0.7 per 10,000 births.

Signs

● Ocular colobomata may affect any of the structures or the entire globe traversed by the fetal fissure from the iris to the optic nerve. It has a variable appearance, depending on the extent and severity of the coloboma.

 ▪ Iris: transillumination defect, heterochromia iridis, and "teardrop" pupil (**Fig. 1-9A**)

 ▪ Lens: defect or flattening of lens or absence of lens zonules inferiorly

 ▪ Chorioretina: thinning of the choriocapillaris; pigment clumping along the line of optic fissure closure; colobomatous defect usually with sharp edges and circumscribed by irregular pigmentation; white sclera is seen through defect if all layers of chorioretina are absent; floor of defect sometimes bulges, forming staphyloma

 ▪ Leukocoria: if the uveal defect is large

 ▪ Optic nerve: enlarged, excavated, vertically oval; retinal vessels may radiate in a spoke-like fashion from the nerve (**Fig. 1-9B and C**)

 ▪ Globe: microphthalmia in some cases

 ▪ Vision: ranges from normal to no light perception

● May be associated with a variety of other developmental defects

Differential Diagnosis

● Atypical coloboma
● Retinal toxoplasmosis
● Optic nerve pits
● Morning glory syndrome
● Optic nerve hypoplasia

Diagnostic Evaluation

● Clinical examination of the eye

Treatment

● Patching for amblyopia: if unilateral with optic nerve involvement to stimulate as much potential vision as possible

● Treat ocular complications: cataract, subretinal neovascularization, and retinal breaks or detachment

Prognosis

● Vision depends on involvement of the optic nerve, macula, and papulomacular bundle.

However, visual acuity cannot be predicted from either coloboma size or optic nerve involvement because patients with large colobomata with optic nerve involvement can have almost normal vision.

REFERENCES

Chang L, Blain D, Bertuzzi S, et al. Uveal coloboma: clinical and basic science update. *Curr Opin Ophthalmol.* 2006;17:447–470.

Onwochei BC, Simon JW, Bateman JB, et al. Ocular colobomata. *Surv Ophthalmol.* 2000;45:175–194.

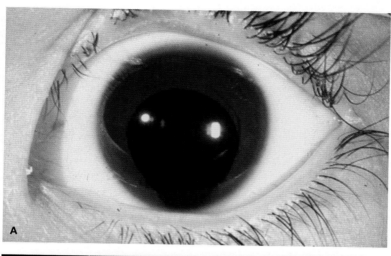

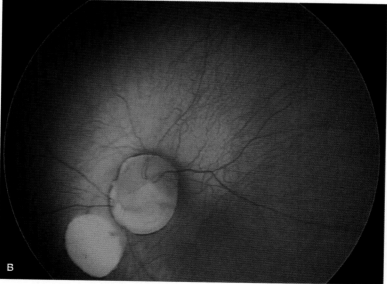

FIGURE 1-9. Coloboma. **A.** Iris coloboma. **B.** Coloboma involving the retina and optic nerve showing an enlarged optic nerve and radiating retinal vessels.

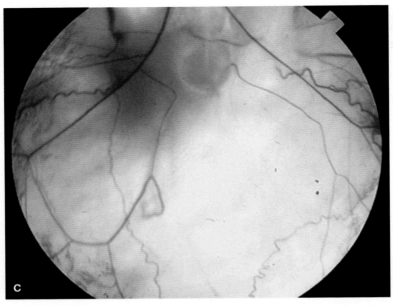

FIGURE 1-9. (*continued*) **C.** Extensive chorioretinal and optic nerve coloboma. Note the round, yellow-appearing optic nerve and the significant disorganization of the tissues.

Congenital Corneal Opacity

Bruce M. Schnall and Michael J. Bartiss ■

The differential diagnosis for congenital corneal opacity can be remembered using the mnemonic STUMPED:

Sclerocornea

Tears in Descemet membrane or birth trauma

Ulcer or infection

Mucopolysaccharidosis (MPS)

Peters anomaly

Endothelial dystrophy, congenital hereditary (CHED)

Dermoid

SCLEROCORNEA

Etiology

- Developmental anomaly of the cornea
- Defective mesodermal migration during embryogenesis, resulting in tissue resembling sclera rather than clear corneal stroma
- Can be autosomal dominant, recessive, or sporadic
- Has been associated with the 22q11.2 deletion syndrome

Symptoms

- Opacified cornea present since birth

Signs

- Usually bilateral but can be unilateral
- Opacification of the cornea with the peripheral cornea more opacified than the central cornea (**Fig. 2-1**)
- May have fine blood vessels

Differential Diagnosis

- Tears in Descemet membrane or birth trauma
- Ulcer or infection
- MPS
- Peters anomaly
- CHED
- Dermoid
- Glaucoma

Treatment

- Evaluation by a genetic specialist to look for associated congenital anomalies
- If the central cornea is clear, it can be associated with cornea plana and a high refractive error.

- Penetrating keratoplasty should be considered if the central visual axis is involved and the posterior segment is relatively normal.

Prognosis

- Visual outcome with or without keratoplasty depends on the presence of other ocular and systemic abnormalities.

REFERENCES

Binenbaum G, McDonald-McGinn DM, Zackai EH, et al. Sclerocornea associated with the chromosome 22q11.2 deletion syndrome. *Am J Med Genet A.* 2008;146(7):904–909.

Doane JF, Sajjadi H, Richardson WP. Bilateral penetrating keratoplasty for sclerocornea in an infant with monosomy 21. Case report and review of the literature. *Cornea.* 1994;13(5):454–458.

Kim T, Cohen EJ, Schnall BM, et al. Ultrasound biomicroscopy and histopathology of sclerocornea. *Cornea.* 1998;17(4):443–445.

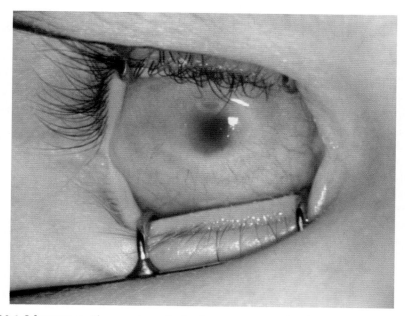

FIGURE 2-1. **Sclerocornea.** The corneal opacification is more severe peripherally than centrally.

BIRTH TRAUMA: TEARS IN DESCEMET MEMBRANE

Etiology

• Trauma to the cornea during vaginal delivery resulting in tears in Descemet membrane

• May be associated with the use of forceps

Symptoms

• Corneal edema or opacification present at birth, which may resolve within the first few days of life

Signs

• Unilateral corneal edema or opacification present at birth (Fig. 2-2A)

• Often observed to have eyelid swelling and evidence of trauma to eyelids at birth

• Corneal edema often resolves within the first few days of life, revealing the Descemet membrane ruptures, which usually appear as vertical linear tears (Fig. 2-2B and C). Descemet tears associated with congenital glaucoma are usually oriented horizontally or curvilinearly (Fig. 2-3).

• Multiple tears are often present.

• Associated with high astigmatism

Differential Diagnosis

• Sclerocornea

• Ulcer or infection

• MPS

• Peters anomaly

• CHED

• Dermoid

• Glaucoma

Treatment

• Descemet tears are associated with high astigmatism, which is amblyogenic. Treatment of the amblyopia includes correction of the refractive error with glasses or contacts and part-time occlusion of the fellow eye.

• Penetrating keratoplasty should be considered if the corneal edema does not resolve.

Prognosis

• Visual outcome depends on the success of amblyopia treatment.

REFERENCE

Lambert SR, Drack AV, Hutchinson AK. Longitudinal changes in the refractive errors of children with tears in Descemet's membrane following forceps injuries. *J AAPOS.* 2004;8(4):368–370.

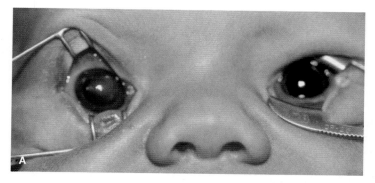

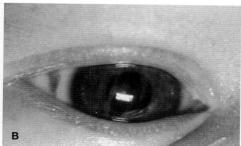

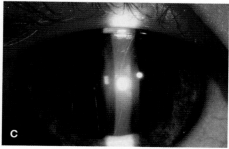

FIGURE 2-2. Descemet tears due to birth trauma. A. Corneal opacification in a newborn from Descemet tears associated with birth trauma. **B.** The vertically oriented linear Descemet membrane ruptures can now be seen in the same infant a few days later after the corneal edema has cleared. **C.** The vertically oriented Descemet membrane breaks from birth trauma can be seen in this older child at the slit lamp with retroillumination.

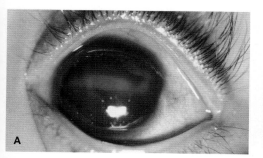

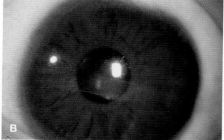

FIGURE 2-3. Descemet tears due to congenital glaucoma. A. Recent Descemet membrane ruptures associated with glaucoma. Note that the breaks are oriented horizontally. They are recent and therefore have overlying corneal edema. **B.** Breaks in Descemet membrane caused by glaucoma. The horizontally oriented breaks can be seen more clearly after resolution of the corneal edema.

ULCER OR INFECTION

Etiology

- Acquired bacterial or herpetic infection

Symptoms

- Acquired corneal opacity usually associated with conjunctival injection and eyelid swelling (Fig. 2-4)

Signs

- Usually unilateral

- Corneal opacity with overlying epithelial defect

- Associated with conjunctival injection and other signs of inflammation

- May have associated systemic infection

- May have associated eyelid lesions or eyelid abnormalities

Differential Diagnosis

- Sclerocornea
- Tears in Descemet membrane from birth trauma
- MPS
- Peters anomaly
- CHED
- Dermoid
- Glaucoma

Treatment

- Depends on underlying cause or organism
- Prompt systemic treatment may be needed.

Prognosis

- May result in a visually significant corneal scar

REFERENCE

Luchs JI, Laibson PR, Stefanyszyn MA, et al. Infantile ulcerative keratitis secondary to congenital entropion. *Cornea.* 1997;16:1:32–34.

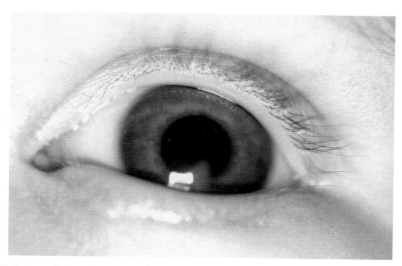

FIGURE 2-4. Corneal ulceration. Corneal ulcer in an infant caused by congenital entropion of the lower eyelid.

MUCOPOLYSACCHARIDOSIS

Etiology

- Inborn error of metabolism
- Enzyme deficiency leads to a block in the metabolic pathway, which results in accumulation of material in the cornea.

Symptoms

- Acquired opacification of the cornea:
  - Hurler syndrome, or MPS 1H, is associated with corneal clouding by 6 months of age.
  - Scheie syndrome, or MPS 1S, is associated with corneal clouding by 12 to 24 months of age.

Signs

- Acquired corneal cloudiness or haze (**Fig. 2-5**)
- Associated systemic features (coarse facial features, mental retardation, poor growth, deafness)

Differential Diagnosis

- Sclerocornea
- Tears in Descemet membrane or birth trauma
- Ulcer or infection
- Peters anomaly
- CHED
- Dermoid
- Glaucoma

Diagnosis

- Evaluation by a genetic specialist
- Urine testing for MPS
- Enzyme assay
- Gene testing for gene defect

Treatment

- Enzyme replacement
- Bone marrow transplant

Prognosis

- Depends on severity of systemic disease and success of systemic treatment

REFERENCE

Kenyon KR, Navon SE, Haritoglou C. Corneal manifestations of metabolic diseases. In: Krachmer JH, Mannis MJ, Hollane EJ, eds. *Cornea*. 2nd ed. Vol 1. Philadelphia, PA: Elsevier Mosby; 2005:749–776.

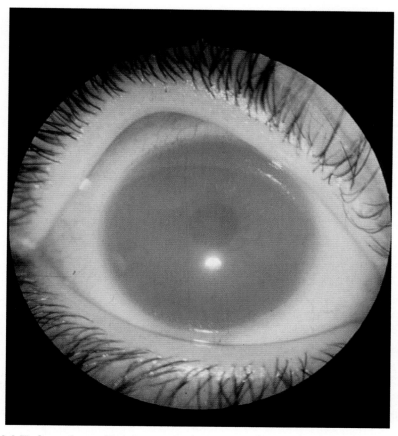

FIGURE 2-5. **Hurler syndrome.** Note the generalized corneal haze. (Courtesy of Alex Levin, MD.)

PETERS ANOMALY

Etiology

- Congenital
- Can be autosomal dominant, recessive, or sporadic
- May be associated with mutation of the *PAX6* gene

Symptoms

- Central corneal opacity present at birth (Fig. 2-6)
- Eighty percent are bilateral.

Signs

- Central corneal leukoma with adherent iris strands (Fig. 2-7)
- Adherent iris strands usually originate from the iris collarette to the posterior surface of the corneal leukoma.
- May have associated cataract and glaucoma

Differential Diagnosis

- Sclerocornea
- Tears in Descemet membrane or birth trauma
- Ulcer or infection
- MPS
- CHED
- Dermoid
- Glaucoma

Diagnosis

- Examination under anesthesia may be needed to confirm diagnosis and rule out glaucoma.

Treatment

- Evaluation by a genetic specialist to look for associated anomalies and to rule out Peters plus syndrome
- Treat glaucoma if present.
- Penetrating keratoplasty should be considered within the first few months of life if the central visual axis is involved and the posterior segment is relatively normal.
- If a visually significant cataract is present, cataract removal may be needed.

Prognosis

- Depends on involvement of the anterior segment; prognosis is poorer if a cataract or glaucoma is present.
- Depends on success of amblyopia treatment
- Early keratoplasty may reduce amblyopia.

REFERENCES

Mailette De Buy Wenniger-Prick LJ, Hennekam RC. The Peters' plus syndrome: A review. *Ann Genet.* 2002;45(2):97–103.

Yang LL, Lambert SR, Drews-Botsch C, et al. Long-term visual outcome of penetrating keratoplasty in infants and children with Peters anomaly. *J AAPOS.* 2009;13(2):175–180.

Yang LL, Lambert SR, Lynn MJ, et al. Long-term results of corneal graft survival in infants and children with Peters anomaly. *Ophthalmology.* 1999;106(4):833–848.

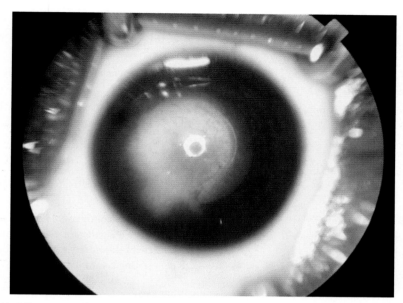

FIGURE 2-6. **Peters anomaly.** Note the central opacity and the clear corneal periphery.

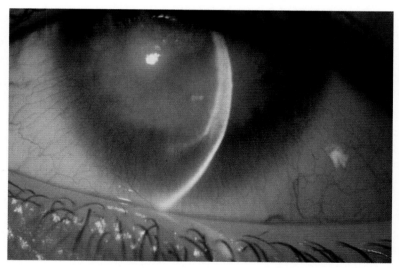

FIGURE 2-7. **Peters anomaly.** Slit-lamp photograph of Peters anomaly. Note the iris adherent to the central corneal leukoma. (Courtesy of Alex Levin, MD.)

CONGENITAL HEREDITARY ENDOTHELIAL DYSTROPHY

Etiology

- Congenital
- Can be autosomal dominant, recessive, or sporadic

Symptoms

- Corneal haze present since birth (Fig. 2-8)

Signs

- Bilateral symmetrical corneal edema
- Swollen, thickened cornea with minimal epithelial edema
- Rarely associated with glaucoma

Differential Diagnosis

- Sclerocornea
- Tears in Descemet membrane from birth trauma
- Ulcer or infection
- MPS
- Peters anomaly
- Dermoid
- Glaucoma

Diagnosis

- CHED can be confused with congenital glaucoma.
- Corneal thickness two to three times normal
- Examination under anesthesia may be needed to confirm corneal thickening and to rule out glaucoma.

Treatment

- Mild edema can be treated with hypertonic saline solutions.
- Penetrating keratoplasty is usually needed if corneal haze is significant. Descemet stripping endothelial keratoplasty may be an alternative to penetrating keratoplasty.

Prognosis

- Depends on graft survival and amblyopia
- Early keratoplasty may reduce amblyopia.

REFERENCES

Javadi MA, Baradaran-Rafii AR, Zamani M, et al. Penetrating keratoplasty in young children with congenital hereditary endothelial dystrophy. *Cornea*. 2003;22(5):420–423.

Mittal V, Mittal R, Sangwan VS. Successful Descemet stripping endothelial keratoplasty in congenital hereditary endothelial dystrophy. *Cornea*. 201;30(3):354–656.

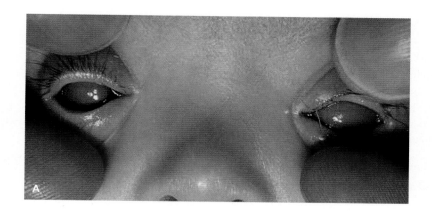

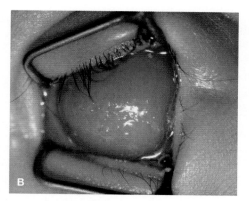

FIGURE 2-8. **Congenital hereditary endothelial dystrophy.** (Courtesy of Alex Levin, MD.)

CORNEAL DERMOID

Etiology

- Developmental anomaly of the cornea
- Limbal dermoids may be associated with Goldenhar syndrome, also known as facio-auricular vertebral syndrome and oculo-auriculo-vertebral dysplasia.

Symptoms

- Corneal opacity present since birth

Signs

- Dome-like mass of the cornea
- Most commonly located at the corneal limbus (epibulbar dermoid) but can be located centrally (Fig. 2-9)
- May contain hairs or fatty tissue (lipodermoids)
- Normal intraocular pressure (IOP) and corneal diameter

Differential Diagnosis

- Sclerocornea
- Tears in Descemet membrane from birth trauma
- Ulcer or infection
- MPS
- Peters anomaly
- CHED
- Glaucoma

Treatment

- Often associated with astigmatism, which will result in amblyopia
- Patching and correction of refractive error may be needed to treat amblyopia.
- Some corneal or limbal dermoids can be treated by shaving flush with corneal surface or lamellar keratoplasty.
- Penetrating keratoplasty can be considered if the central visual axis is involved.

Prognosis

- Visual outcome depends on success of amblyopia treatment.

REFERENCES

Arora R, Jain V, Mehta D. Deep lamellar keratoplasty in corneal dermoid. *Eye (Lond)*. 2005;19(8):920–921.

Mansour AM, Barber JC, Reinecke RD, et al. Ocular choristomas. *Surv Ophthalmol*. 1989;33(5):339–358.

Watts P, Michaeli-Cohen A, Abdolell M, et al. Outcome of lamellar keratoplasty for limbal dermoids in children. *J AAPOS*. 2002;6(4):209–215.

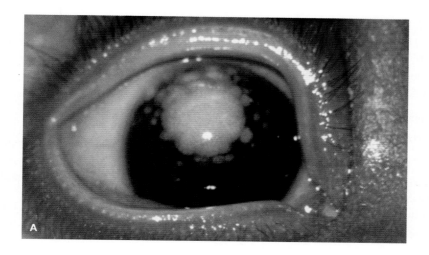

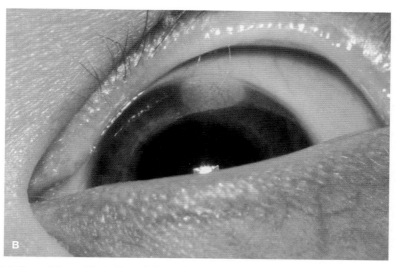

FIGURE 2-9. Corneal dermoid. A. Centrally located corneal dermoid. Note the satellite-like lesions. **B.** Dermoid located at the limbus superiorly.

ANTERIOR STAPHYLOMA

Etiology

- Developmental anomaly of the anterior segment

Symptoms

- Bulging opacified cornea

Signs

- Bulging or protuberant congenital corneal opacity that may prevent the eyelids from closing fully
- Can be unilateral or bilateral (Fig. 2-10)
- Cornea usually thinned and enlarged

Differential Diagnosis

- Sclerocornea
- Tears in Descemet membrane from birth trauma
- Ulcer or infection
- MPS
- Peters anomaly
- CHED
- Dermoid

Treatment

- Often treated with evisceration or enucleation (Fig. 2-11)
- Corneoscleral transplant can be considered.

Prognosis

- Visual prognosis is poor.

REFERENCE

Lunardelli P, Matayoshi S. Congenital anterior staphyloma. *J Pediatr Ophthalmol Strabismus.* 2009;25:1–2.

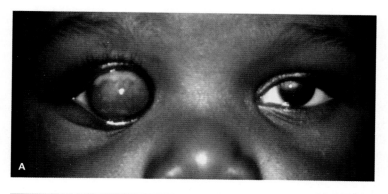

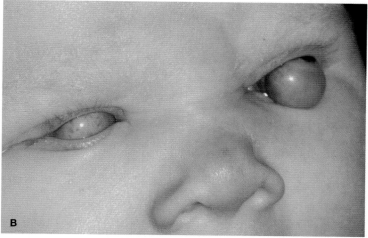

FIGURE 2-10. **Anterior staphyloma.** **A.** Unilateral anterior staphyloma. **B.** Bilateral anterior staphyloma.

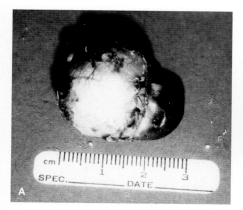

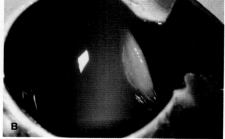

FIGURE 2-11. **Enucleation specimen of anterior staphyloma.** **A.** Gross specimen of enucleated eye with anterior staphyloma; note the bulging cornea. **B.** Specimen showing view of lens and anterior staphyloma to the right of the lens.

WILSON DISEASE (HEPATOLENTICULAR DEGENERATION)

Etiology

- Autosomal recessive inherited disorder caused by multiple allelic substitutions or deletions in the DNA coding for B-polypeptide, Cu^{++} transporting, and ATPase
- Defect linked to chromosome 13q14.3-q21.1
- Systemic decreased level of ceruloplasmin causing decreased ability to properly transport copper
- Copper deposition in liver and kidneys followed by brain and Descemet membrane

Symptoms

- Muscular rigidity, tremor, and involuntary movements (can resemble Parkinson disease)
- Speech difficulties and dementia also occur.

Signs

- Golden brown, red, or green ring of pigmentation (known as Kayser-Fleischer ring) at the level of the posterior lamella of Descemet membrane (Fig. 2-12)
- Usually begin at the 12- and 6-o'clock positions in the cornea and spread circumferentially around the cornea
- May be several millimeters thick

Differential Diagnosis

- Intrahepatic cholestasis of childhood
- Biliary cirrhosis
- Chronic active hepatitis

Treatment

Kayser-Fleischer rings gradually disappear with successful treatment.

- D-penicillamine (works via chelating Cu^{++} ions)
- British anti-Lewisite
- Copper-deficient diet
- Liver transplantation

Prognosis

- Studies have shown retinal electrophysiologic abnormalities improving with successful treatment.

REFERENCES

Liu M, Cohen EJ, Brewer GJ, Laibson PR. Kayser-Fleischer ring as the presenting sign of Wilson disease. *Am J Ophthalmol.* 2002;133(6):832–834.

Slovis TL, Dubois RS, Rodgerson DO, Silverman A. The varied manifestations of Wilson's disease. *J Pediatr.* 1971;78(4):578–584.

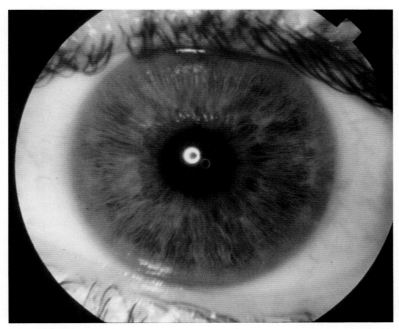

FIGURE 2-12. Wilson disease. Kayser-Fleisher ring in a patient with Wilson disease. Note the brown-red ring in the periphery of the cornea.

HERPES SIMPLEX INFECTION

Etiology

- Infection with herpes simplex virus (HSV) type 1 or 2
- Usually acquired during childhood, occasionally acquired during the birth process
- Ocular infection with HSV can affect the eyelids, conjunctiva, or cornea.
- HSV blepharoconjunctivitis

Symptoms

- Vesicular lesions on the eyelid or red inflamed eye
- Vesicles cross the dermatomes and progress to crusting (Fig. 2-13).
- Usually unilateral
- May be recurrent

Signs

- Clear vesicles with an erythematous base
- Often associated with an enlarged preauricular lymph node on the affected side

- Conjunctival involvement results in conjunctival injection and eyelid swelling.
- May be associated with a conjunctival dendrite, which is best seen at the slit lamp with fluorescein

Differential Diagnosis

- Herpes zoster ophthalmicus: Rash is dermatomal and does not cross the midline.

Diagnosis

- Based on characteristic clinical findings
- In atypical cases, diagnosis can be confirmed by viral cultures, polymerase chain reaction (PCR) testing, or the appearance of multinucleated giant cells on Giemsa staining of scrapings.

Treatment

- Topical (trifluridine drops or ganciclovir ophthalmic gel) or systemic (acyclovir or valacyclovir) antiviral agents (or both topical and systemic agents) may be used.
- Long-term oral antiviral prophylaxis is recommended for children with multiple recurrent episodes.

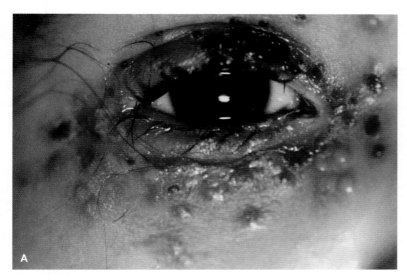

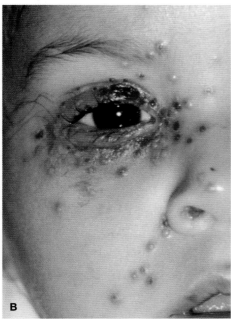

FIGURE 2-13. Herpes simplex blepharitis.
A. Vesicular lesions, some of which are now crusted. **B.** The vesicular lesions cross dermatomes.

HERPES SIMPLEX VIRUS EPITHELIAL DENDRITE OR ULCERATION

Symptoms

- Red, painful eye
- Tearing, photophobia, decreased vision
- History of previous HSV infection
- Usually unilateral

Signs

- Dendrite that appears as a linear branching epithelial defect with terminal bulbs (Fig. 2-14A)
- May appear as a geographic ulceration (Fig. 2-14B)
- Epithelial edges of herpetic lesions are swollen and stain intensely

Diagnosis

- Based on characteristic clinical findings
- In atypical cases, diagnosis can be confirmed by viral cultures, PCR testing, or the appearance of multinucleated giant cells on Giemsa staining of corneal scrapings.

Treatment

- Topical (trifluridine drops or ganciclovir ophthalmic gel) or systemic (acyclovir or valacyclovir) antiviral agents (or both topical and systemic agents) may be used
- Consider cycloplegics for significant photophobia or uveitis if present.
- Debridement can remove infected epithelium.

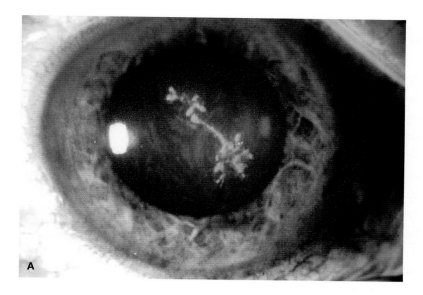

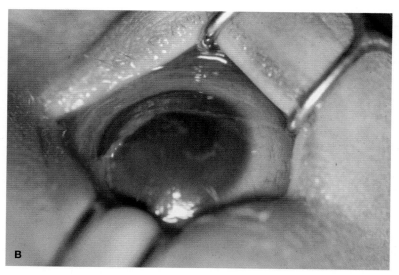

FIGURE 2-14. Herpes simplex virus epithelilal disease. A. Herpes simplex corneal dendrite. The dendrite stains with fluorescein when viewed with cobalt blue light. (Courtesy of Alex Levin, MD.) **B.** Herpes simplex geographic corneal ulcer in an infant. Note the white, raised leading edge of the ulcer.

HERPES SIMPLEX VIRUS CORNEAL STROMAL DISEASE

Symptoms

- Unilateral corneal opacity (Fig. 2-15)
- Red, painful eye
- Tearing, photophobia, decreased vision
- History of previous HSV infection

Signs

- Disciform keratitis (Fig. 2-16A)
  - Disc-shaped stromal opacity
  - Intact epithelium
  - Mild anterior chamber reaction
  - Keratoprecipitates are common.
- Interstitial keratitis (Fig. 2-16B)
  - Multiple or diffuse white stromal infiltrates
  - Neovascularization or ghost vessels

Diagnosis

- Based on characteristic clinical findings
- Decreased corneal sensation

Treatment

- Combination of antiviral agents and steroids

REFERENCES

Chong EM, Wilhelmus KR, Matoba AY, et al. Herpes simplex virus keratitis in children. *Am J Ophthalmol.* 2004;138(3):474–475.

Hsiao CH, Yeung L, Yeh LK, et al. Pediatric herpes simplex virus keratitis. *Cornea.* 2009;28(3):249–253.

Schwartz GS, Holland EJ. Oral acyclovir for the management of herpes simplex virus keratitis in children. *Ophthalmology.* 2000;107(2):278–282.

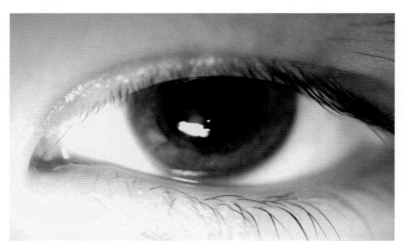

FIGURE 2-15. Herpes simplex virus stromal disease.   Corneal opacity in an uninflamed eye months after herpes simplex infection.

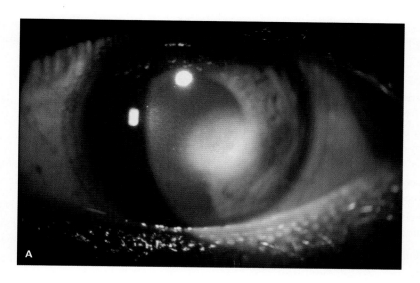

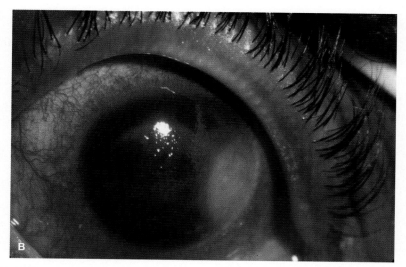

FIGURE 2-16. Herpes simplex virus stromal disease. **A.** Active herpes simplex interstitial keratitis. **B.** Disciform keratitis. Note the disc-like corneal haze seen in the slit-lamp photograph.

HERPES ZOSTER OPHTHALMICUS

Etiology

- Reactivation of latent varicella (chickenpox virus) from cranial nerve ganglia
- More common in the elderly population but may occur if the child had chickenpox in utero or within the first 6 months of life
- Has occurred in children immunized for chickenpox
- Can occur in individuals who are immunocompromised

Symptoms

- Unilateral vesicular lesions associated with pain
- May be preceded by headache or neuralgia in affected dermatome

Signs

- Vesicular rash isolated to the dermatome of the fifth cranial nerve (Fig. 2-17)
- Rash usually respects the midline
- May develop conjunctivitis, small epithelial dendrites (pseudodendrites), disciform keratitis, and uveitis
- Corneal disease and uveitis may not begin until several days to weeks after the onset of the skin eruption.

Differential Diagnosis

- Herpes simplex: Rash is not dermatomal and crosses the midline.

Diagnosis

- Based on characteristic clinical findings and associated skin vesicles

Treatment

- Systemic antivirals are recommended within 4 days of onset of skin eruptions.
- Analgesics may be needed to treat associated pain.
- Conjunctivitis and pseudodendrites can be treated with lubrication.
- Disciform keratitis and uveitis are treated with topical steroids.

REFERENCE

De Freitas D, Martins EN, Adan C, et al. Herpes zoster ophthalmicus in otherwise healthy children. *Am J Ophthalmol.* 2006;142(3):393–399.

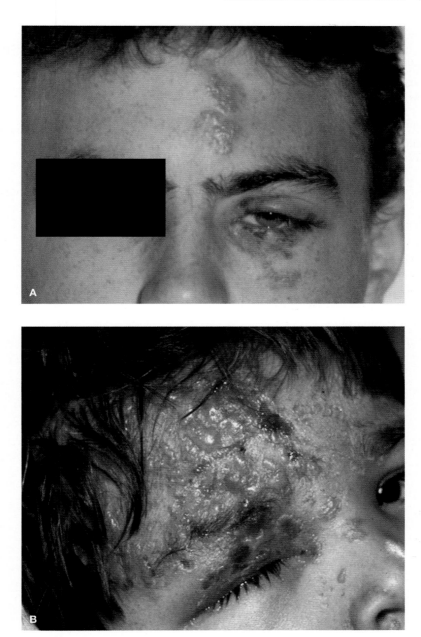

FIGURE 2-17. Herpes zoster ophthalmicus. Note the dermatomal distribution of the vesicles (**A** and **B**) and the significant eyelid edema (**B**).

CHICKENPOX

Etiology

- Primary infection with varicella (chickenpox virus)

Symptoms

- Disseminated vesicular lesions that affect the skin and mucous membranes
- Red eye, conjunctival lesion (Fig. 2-18)

Signs

- Conjunctival vesicle or ulceration
- Less commonly may develop superficial punctate keratitis, dendrite without terminal bulbs, or disciform keratitis
- Often associated with a transient mild anterior uveitis but can trigger a persistent uveitis that requires treatment

Diagnosis

- Based on characteristic clinical findings and associated skin vesicles

Treatment

- Self-limited conjunctivitis
- Topical antibiotics may prevent secondary bacterial infection.

Prognosis

- Usually resolves without conjunctival or corneal scarring

REFERENCE

Pavan-Langston D. In: Smolin G, Thoft RA, eds. *The Cornea.* Boston, MA: Little, Brown and Company; 1983:189.

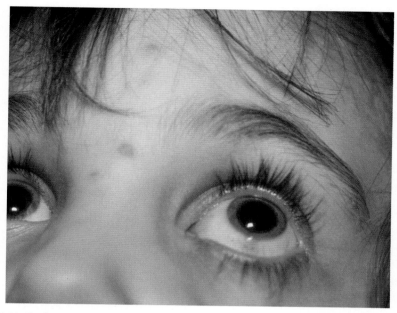

FIGURE 2-18. Chicken pox. Chickenpox lesion can be seen just inferior to the cornea in the left eye and on the face.

LIMBAL VERNAL KERATOCONJUNCTIVITIS

Etiology

- Most common cause is seasonal allergies.

Symptoms

- Elevated gelatinous mass along the corneal limbus
- Red, itchy eyes
- Mucous production

Signs

- Discrete gray-white nodules at cornea limbus. These nodules have a whitish center that is filled with eosinophils (Horner-Trantas dots; Fig. 2-19).
- The nodules may become confluent.
- Conjunctiva surrounding these nodules is injected.
- Usually bilateral, but involvement may be asymmetrical

Diagnosis

- Based on characteristic clinical findings
- History of seasonal allergies

Treatment

- Topical antihistamine and mast cell stabilizers
- Topical steroids may be needed; best used in pulsed doses. When using topical steroids, careful monitoring, including monitoring IOP, is needed to prevent steroid side effects.
- Oral antihistamines and removal of suspected allergens can be helpful.

REFERENCE

Krachmer JH, Mannis MJ, Hollane EJ, eds. *Cornea*. 2nd ed. Vol 1. Philadelphia, PA: Elsevier Mosby; 2005:552–558.

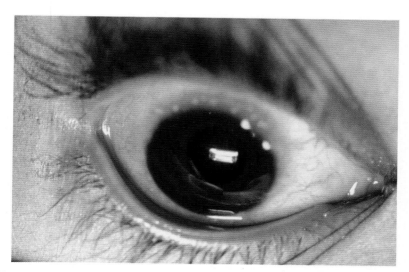

FIGURE 2-19. Limbal vernal. White, elevated lesions (Horner-Trantas dots) can be seen along the corneal limbus superiorly.

Glaucoma

Alex V. Levin and Anya A. Trumler ■

PRIMARY CONGENITAL GLAUCOMA

Glaucoma diagnosed within the first 4 years of life and not associated with other findings of anterior segment dysgenesis is classified as primary *congenital glaucoma* and is further subdivided into *neonatal onset* (onset ≤ 1 month old), *infantile onset* (>1–24 months old), and *late onset* (> 2 years old). Typical findings include buphthalmos, which is usually characterized by corneal enlargement, Haab striae (breaks in Descemet's membrane), corneal edema, and increasing axial length, with patches of anterior iris insertion on gonioscopy. These patients have no other predisposing factors such as cataract surgery, trauma, or steroid use. Neonatal presentation portends a worse prognosis.

Epidemiology and Etiology

● The incidence varies in different populations of the world, with a reported incidence of 1 in 10,000 in the United States. It has a much higher incidence in Saudi Arabia and the Gypsies of Romania (1 per 2500 and 1 per 1250, respectively), with both populations having a higher rate of consanguinity and allele frequency.

● Mutations in the *CYP1B1* gene (2p21), which encodes a cytochrome P450 protein, are one cause. Two other genes and at least two other loci have been identified. In the Arabic and Gypsy populations, a homozygous mutation in *CYP1B1* has been found in more than 94% of cases, consistent with autosomal recessive inheritance. In isolated cases, and in North America, the frequency of *CYP1B1* mutation decreases to 10% to 15%.

● Congenital glaucoma is a primary goniodysgenesis. The theory of an imperforate membrane (Barkan membrane) over the trabecular meshwork is controversial. Rather, there appears to be a failure of complete neural crest differentiation, resulting in impaired aqueous outflow. Clinically, the angle is characterized on gonioscopy as a flat or patchy high insertion with absence of the angle recess and iris inserting directly on the trabecular meshwork (**Fig. 3-1**).

History

● Primary congenital or infantile glaucoma is bilateral in 75% of cases, which can create a delay in diagnosis because parents may simply believe their child has "beautiful big eyes."

- The classic symptoms include photophobia and epiphora due to corneal stromal or epithelial edema (Fig. 3-2). A "cloudy eye" is often the presenting sign.

- Elevated intraocular pressure (IOP) causes stretching of the cornea with resultant breaks in Descemet's membrane, called Haab striae (Fig. 3-3). Buphthalmos also thins the sclera giving it a blue appearance because of the underlying hue of the uvea.

Signs

- Characteristic findings include optic nerve cupping, corneal enlargement, Haab striae, increasing axial length, and gonioscopic findings (see "Diagnostic Evaluation" section). IOP may be artifactually low in the presence of corneal epithelial edema.

Differential Diagnosis

- Congenital hereditary endothelial dystrophy
- Congenital hereditary stromal dystrophy
- Mucopolysaccharidosis
- Peters anomaly and other causes of sclerocornea
- Keratitis
- Forceps birth trauma
- Megalocornea (X-linked recessive or autosomal recessive)
- Contralateral microphthalmia
- Nasolacrimal duct obstruction

Diagnostic Evaluation

- A patient with corneal clouding, increased corneal diameter, and optic nerve cupping should raise the suspicion for primary congenital glaucoma and prompt further evaluation, if needed, with an examination under anesthesia, including slit-lamp biomicroscopy, corneal pachymetry, corneal diameter measurement, gonioscopy, refraction, axial length measurement, and (if possible) optic nerve photography.

- When measuring IOP under anesthesia, attention should be paid regarding the type of anesthetic agent used. Whereas ketamine increases IOP measurements, halothane lowers IOP, as do other anesthetic agents but to a lesser extent.

- Corneal edema falsely lowers the IOP measurements, whereas stromal edema may stiffen the cornea and cause falsely high measurements. Asymmetry of IOP is also a suggestive indication of an abnormality.

- The normal maximum corneal diameter in an infant younger than 1 year is 11 mm. A corneal diameter greater than 12 mm, asymmetry between the eyes, and significant progression over time are all suggestive of congenital glaucoma.

- Retinoscopy and axial length measurement using immersion A-scan provide objective measurements to suggest increased axial length. The mean axial length at birth is 17 mm and increases to 20 mm by 1 year of age.

Treatment and Prognosis

- Medical management with antiglaucoma medications in primary congenital or infantile glaucoma is used as a temporizing agent, with definitive treatment being surgical.

- Antiglaucoma medications, including carbonic anhydrase inhibitors (both topical and oral), low-dose beta-blockers, and prostaglandins, may be used to clear the cornea for surgical intervention. Brimonidine should not be used in infants younger than 1 year because there is a risk of potentially life-threatening apnea, hypotension, bradycardia, and hypothermia.

- The primary procedure of choice is goniotomy or trabeculotomy depending on the preference of the surgeon and adequate visualization of the anterior chamber angle that is needed for goniotomy. Both have reported short-term success rates of 60% to 90%. Goniotomy has the advantage of leaving the conjunctiva untouched. Endoscopic goniotomy can be performed if the cornea is too cloudy to allow for a standard gonioscopic view. Another procedure that has been popularized is 360-degree trabeculotomy.

- In patients who have a history of failed goniotomy or trabeculotomy, secondary surgical interventions may include goniosurgery on the remaining angle, trabeculectomy, or glaucoma drainage device implantation. Neonatal onset congenital glaucoma more often requires surgery beyond or other than goniotomy or trabeculotomy.

- The goal of primary congenital or infantile glaucoma treatment is more than achieving a normal IOP. More importantly, attaining and maintaining normal visual function is paramount the biggest obstacle to which is amblyopia. Aggressive treatment of refractive error, amblyopia, and visually significant optical opacities are important components to the infant's care. Lifelong follow-up of these patients is needed to monitor for glaucoma progression.

- Optic nerve cupping in infants is reversible and is a hallmark of successful glaucoma management.

REFERENCES

Bejjani BA, Lewis RA, Tomey KF, et al. Mutations in CYP1B1, the gene for cytochrome P4501B1, are the predominant cause of primary congenital glaucoma in Saudi Arabia. *Am J Hum Genet.* 1998;62:325–333.

Chen TC, Chn PP, Francis BA, et al. Pediatric glaucoma surgery: a report by the American Academy of Ophthalmology. *Ophthalmology.* 2014;121:2107–2115.

Taylor RH, Ainsworth JR, Evans AR, et al. The epidemiology of pediatric glaucoma: the Toronto experience. *J AAPOS.* 1999;3:308–315.

Yassin SA, Al-Tamimi E. Surgial outcomes in children with primary congenital glaucoma: a 20-year experience. *Eur J Ophthalmol.* 2016;26(6):581–587.

Zagora SL, Funnell CL, Martin FJ, et al. Primary congenital glaucoma outcomes: lessons from 23 years of follow-up. *Am J Ophthalmol.* 2015;159:788–796.

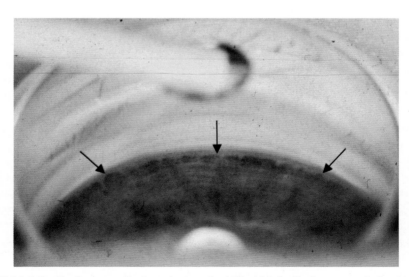

FIGURE 3-1. Infantile glaucoma. Gonioscopic view of a child with infantile glaucoma angle showing patches of high iris insertion (*arrows*).

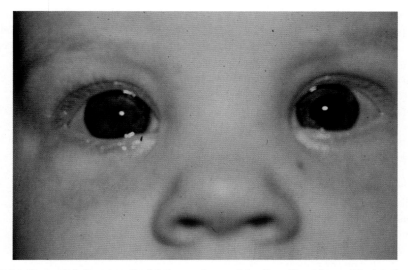

FIGURE 3-2. **Congenital glaucoma.** Buphthalmos and corneal clouding of the right eye. Miosis in the right eye is caused by the use of pilocarpine.

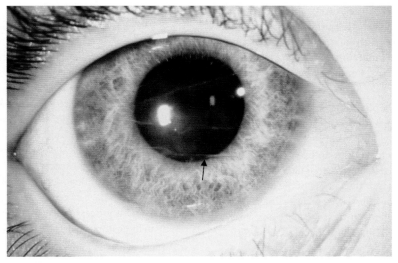

FIGURE 3-3. **Haab striae**, which are breaks in Descemet's membrane, are delineated by the appearance of two scrolled-back edges (*arrows* denote the bottom Haab stria; there is also one more superiorly).

JUVENILE OPEN-ANGLE GLAUCOMA

Juvenile open-angle glaucoma (JOAG) is a form of open-angle primary glaucoma unassociated with ocular malformations or other inciting factors, with an age of onset from 4 to 40 years. JOAG generally has a more aggressive course than the later-onset adult primary open-angle glaucoma.

Epidemiology and Etiology

• The incidence of JOAG is 1 per 50,000 cases of all glaucoma. It has autosomal dominant inheritance with variable expression and penetrance. One known mutated gene is the myocilin gene (*MYOC*) on chromosome 1q21-q31 (termed GLC1A). Myocilin is a glycoprotein that is expressed in the trabecular meshwork, with its function largely unknown. Mutations in the *CYP1B1* gene on chromosome 2p21 have been associated with autosomal recessive inheritance of juvenile onset glaucoma. Patients with a mutation in *CYP1B1* in addition to *MYOC* have a more severe phenotype than those with *MYOC* mutation alone.

• The pathophysiology of JOAG is unknown but is thought to be impaired aqueous outflow through the trabecular meshwork. There are usually no abnormalities on gonioscopy in affected patients, although there are histologic reports of thickening of the trabecular meshwork outflow system and clinical reports of increased iris processes ("pectinate ligaments") crossing the trabecular meshwork.

• Most cases of JOAG that have a strong family history of disease are associated with mutation in *MYOC* and demonstrate an autosomal dominant pattern.

History

• Patients are usually asymptomatic. Often, the disorder is noted as an incidental finding during routine examination.

• Because it is most commonly an autosomal dominant disorder, at-risk family members of affected individuals should have a comprehensive examination.

Signs

• JOAG is an aggressive, usually bilateral, disease that results in optic nerve cupping, visual field changes, and nerve fiber layer thinning in the presence of elevated IOP.

Differential Diagnosis

• Glaucoma associated with acquired conditions

• Glaucoma associated with nonacquired ocular anomalies

• Glaucoma associated with nonacquired systemic disease or syndrome

• Optic atrophy

• Physiologic cupping

Diagnostic Evaluation

• At-risk children based on family history (one affected parent or sibling) should have IOP measurements at least every 6 months even if sedation or anesthesia is required. Evaluation should include a comprehensive ophthalmic examination, including vision, refraction, slit-lamp examination, corneal pachymetry, and ophthalmoscopy. Gonioscopy is not diagnostic but is useful in evaluating for secondary causes of glaucoma. The presence of increased numbers of iris processes may or may not represent an indicator of risk for JOAG.

• Patients with the clinical appearance of glaucomatous optic neuropathy with normal IOP on isolated visits can also undergo diurnal curve testing to assess pressure variation as well as maximum daily pressure.

• Automated visual field testing in young patients can be difficult, with Goldman visual field testing often being an easier if not more reliable assessment tool.

- Optical coherence tomography (OCT) currently has available normative data for children older than 4 years, but asymmetry between the two eyes and changes over time are important indicators of abnormality.

- Optic nerve photography is useful in documenting and monitoring changes in the appearance of the optic nerves.

- Physiologic cupping, also an autosomal dominant condition, must be considered (Fig. 3-4) but is difficult to distinguish from JOAG other than the absence of elevated IOP, change over time, or visual field deficits. Physiologic cups tend to have distinct sharp borders and may be eccentric within the disc. Parents of the proband should be examined for similar findings and, if present, their IOP should be checked as well. It may take several visits over months or years to be confident that there is no progression and thus no JOAG.

Treatment and Prognosis

- JOAG tends to be more aggressive, more resistant to medical therapy, and associated with more severe visual impairment.

- The use of topical antiglaucoma medications is the first line of treatment followed by oral carbonic anhydrase inhibitors.

- JOAG patients require close follow-up until maintenance of an acceptable IOP is achieved.

- Many cases over the long term are progressive and require surgical intervention.

- Some evidence indicates that goniotomy or trabeculotomy can be successful. More traditionally, trabeculectomy or glaucoma drainage device surgery is the first surgical intervention. Trabeculectomy has similar success rates to those done on patients with primary open-angle glaucoma.

REFERENCES

Coppens G, Stalmans I, Zeyren T, Casteels I. The safety and efficacy of glaucoma medications in the pediatric population. *J Pediatr Ophthalmol Strabismus.* 2009;46:12–18.

Park SC, Kee C. Large diurnal variation of intraocular pressure despite maximal medical treatment in juvenile open angle glaucoma. *J Glaucoma.* 2007;16:164–168.

Stoilova D, Child A, Brice G, et al. Novel TIGR/MYOC mutations in families with juvenile onset primary open angle glaucoma. *J Med Genet.* 1998;35:989–992.

Vincent AL, Billingsley G, Buys Y, et al. Digenic inheritance of early-onset glaucoma: CYP1B1, a potential modifier gene. *Am J Hum Genet.* 2002;70:448–460.

Yeung HH, Walton DS. Goniotomy for juvenile open-angle glaucoma. *J Glaucoma.* 2010;19:1–4.

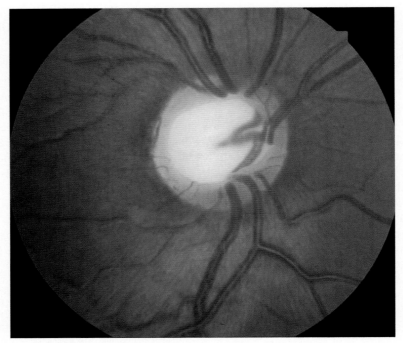

FIGURE 3-4. Physiologic cup. Note the sharp margin to the cup and scooped-out appearance. The vessels disappear as they turn posteriorly at the margin of the cup. The father, who did not have glaucoma, has a similar appearance to his optic nerve heads.

GLAUCOMA FOLLOWING CATARACT SURGERY

All children who have cataract surgery, regardless of whether they are left aphakic or pseudophakic, are at risk for glaucoma. The phrase *glaucoma following cataract surgery* applies to any child who has had cataract surgery and then developed glaucoma, even if they have other preexisting risk factors such as ocular anomalies, uveitis, or steroid use. This category of glaucoma is divided into closed angle if more than 50% of the angle is closed, or open angle.

Epidemiology and Etiology

● Aphakic glaucoma is the most common complication of congenital cataract surgery, with an incidence up to 32%. Theories as to the etiology include abnormal development of the anterior chamber angle, genetic predisposition, barotrauma incurred during surgery, decreased structural support to the drainage angle, vitreous affecting angle structures, and release of chemical mediators through an open posterior capsule that affect aqueous drainage.

● Despite advances in cataract surgery, it is clear that the prevention of glaucoma after cataract surgery has not been well achieved. Even with the use of intraocular lens implantation in the pediatric population, the incidence of glaucoma appears to be unchanged.

● Factors associated with a higher risk of development of glaucoma are surgery within the first year of life, corneal diameter less than 10 mm, presence of other ocular anomalies, retained lens material, nuclear cataract, and eyes that require secondary surgeries.

History

● Similar to primary congenital glaucoma, the symptoms of photophobia, epiphora, and blepharospasm are often seen in those who develop aphakic glaucoma before age 3 years. Older patients are usually asymptomatic.

● The onset of glaucoma may occur early after surgery or later in childhood, with the average age to onset approximately 4 to 8 years after surgery.

● Routine lifelong screening of all children who have had cataract surgery is important for the early diagnosis of glaucoma.

Signs

● Early signs of glaucoma include a decrease in the amount of rapid loss of hyperopia caused by globe elongation, corneal clouding, increased corneal diameter, and even Haab stria in patients who develop glaucoma generally before age 3 years.

● Most patients are asymptomatic, and elevated IOP and optic nerve cupping are found on screening examination.

● The presence of peripheral or midperipheral anterior synechia or posterior synechia with iris bombe speaks to an inflammatory component.

Differential Diagnosis

● Primary congenital glaucoma

● Glaucoma associated with acquired conditions

● Glaucoma associated with nonacquired ocular anomalies

● Glaucoma associated with nonacquired systemic disease or syndrome

Diagnostic Evaluation

● Pediatric patients who have had cataract surgery should be examined for glaucoma on a regular basis, certainly no less than annually. When patients are too young for IOP measurement or optic nerve evaluation, an examination under anesthesia or sedation may be needed.

● Early signs of glaucoma include a decrease in the amount of aphakic refraction, corneal clouding, increased corneal diameter in young patients, and optic nerve cupping.

- Ultrasound biomicroscopy, corneal pachymetry (which is often elevated in aphakia and pseudophakia), and gonioscopy may offer information that is useful in diagnosis and management. Gonioscopy may show an angle configuration similar to that seen in primary infantile glaucoma (Fig. 3-5), a closed angle, or peripheral anterior synechia.

- Axial length measurement, OCT, and optic nerve photography are all important tools to monitor the disease.

Treatment and Prognosis

- The first line of treatment of patients with aphakic glaucoma is one or more antiglaucoma medications, which in many cases prove effective in lowering the IOP.

- When topical and oral medications fail, surgery is often successful, with goniotomy or trabeculotomy being effective in approximately 55% of patients, usually those that have an angle configuration similar to that seen in primary congenital glaucoma.

- Trabeculectomy or glaucoma drainage device may be used. Endoscopic diode cyclophotoablation may provide another early option for treatment. Otherwise, cycloablation plays a role only in cases of refractive glaucoma.

- Early detection and treatment of glaucoma are important in improving the likelihood of preventing optic nerve progression and preserving visual function.

- Aggressive treatment of refractive error, amblyopia, and visually significant optical opacities are also vital components of obtaining the best vision outcomes.

REFERENCES

Bothun ED, Guo Y, Christiansen SP, et al. Outcome of angle surgery in children with aphakic glaucoma. *J AAPOS.* 2010;14:235–239.

Chen TC, Walton DS, Bhatia LS. Aphakic glaucoma after congenital cataract surgery. *Arch Ophthalmol.* 2004;122:1819–1825.

Levin AV. Aphakic glaucoma: a never-ending story? *Br J Ophthalmol.* 2007;91:1574–1575.

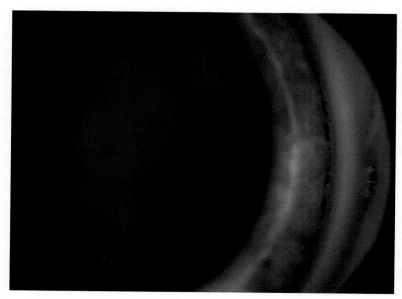

FIGURE 3-5. **Aphakic glaucoma.** Gonioscopy of the angle in aphakic glaucoma appears similar to infantile glaucoma with patches of high iris insertion. This patient may be a good candidate for goniolytic surgery.

UVEITIC GLAUCOMA

Glaucoma due to uveitis is a form of *glaucoma associated with acquired conditions* and can be further divided into those with open angle (≥50% open) and closed angle.

Epidemiology and Etiology

• The prevalence of pediatric uveitis is 30 cases per 100,000. Over a 5-year follow-up period, 35% of all children with uveitis have an episode of elevated IOP.

• Uveitis is associated with an increased risk of glaucoma not only because of the underlying process of uveitis but also because of the long-term use of corticosteroid treatments. However, the risk of glaucoma from untreated uveitis is far greater than the risk of steroids.

• The pathophysiology of uveitis inducing glaucoma is complex. In uveitis, vascular permeability is increased in the ciliary body, which results in aqueous hypersecretion and increased protein content. There is an increase in aqueous prostaglandins, which increases uveoscleral outflow at low concentrations but decreases uveoscleral outflow at higher concentrations.

• Aqueous outflow through the trabecular meshwork can be decreased by inflammatory cells and fibrin in the angle. Uveitis may also induce swelling or dysfunction of the trabecular meshwork and trabecular endothelium, decreasing outflow (trabeculitis).

• Peripheral anterior synechiae form in uveitis, with the most severe cases resulting in angle-closure glaucoma.

• Posterior synechia can result in pupillary block with iris bombe (see Fig. 3-6).

• Chronic inflammation and ischemia can lead to neovascular glaucoma.

• Although glaucoma can occur in every type of uveitis, certain etiologies of uveitis have a higher incidence, particularly juvenile idiopathic arthritis (JIA). Posterior uveitis has a lower risk of inducing glaucoma than anterior uveitis.

History

• Acute anterior uveitis is characterized by photophobia, pain, redness, decreased vision, and epiphora except for children with JIA who are usually asymptomatic until late in the disease when they may present with irregularity of the pupil, band keratopathy, or decreased vision from cataracts, inflammation, and posterior synechiae.

• In posterior uveitis, the only symptoms may be floaters and blurred vision.

• Glaucoma is asymptomatic unless an acute significant elevation in IOP occurs as may be seen with pupillary block due to posterior synechia.

• In patients with uveitis, it is important to obtain a thorough history, including past medical history and review of symptoms along with appropriate laboratory testing to try to determine the etiology of the inflammation and thus improve management.

Signs

• Slit-lamp examination is useful to quantify the amount of inflammation, assess peripheral and central anterior chamber depth, and diagnose the presence of posterior synechiae and neovascularization.

• Peripheral anterior synechiae can be visualized on gonioscopy. The extent of peripheral anterior synechiae is not diagnostic for glaucoma but is a risk factor.

• As in all forms of glaucoma, optic nerve evaluation is important in diagnosing and monitoring disease progression.

• Diagnostic tests such as OCT and visual fields become more difficult because media opacities are more likely to be present in patients with uveitis.

Differential Diagnosis

- Other causes of glaucoma associated with acquired conditions include:
  - Steroid-induced glaucoma
  - Angle-closure glaucoma
  - Tumor (masquerade syndrome, e.g., leukemia, retinoblastoma)
  - Ghost cell glaucoma following hemorrhage
  - Traumatic glaucoma

Diagnostic Evaluation

- As in all cases of uveitis, the extent of ocular involvement is determined by a comprehensive ophthalmic examination.

- Despite active or inactive disease, continued monitoring for glaucoma is imperative.

- On slit-lamp biomicroscopy, the examination of the anterior segment includes cornea for keratoprecipitates, band keratopathy and epithelial dendrites, anterior chamber depth, and evaluation for cells and flare; examination of the iris for stromal atrophy, nodules, posterior synechiae, and peripheral anterior synechiae; and examination of the lens for cataract.

- IOP should be checked in all patients with uveitis during every visit if possible.

- Shallowing of the anterior chamber, increased IOP, and peripheral anterior synechiae are indications for performing gonioscopy if possible.

- Dilation with thorough examination of the posterior segment is necessary to help determine the extent as well as the cause of the uveitis. The optic nerve appearance should also be monitored for changes of glaucomatous optic neuropathy.

- In patients with acute uveitis and healthy optic nerves, transient elevated IOP might be monitored because a decrease may occur with aggressive treatment of the inflammation. Chronic and recurrent uveitis with elevated IOP or at-risk nerves requires a lower threshold for treatment.

- A steroid-related increase in IOP rarely occurs within 2 weeks of initiating treatment, but the clearance of protein and cells from the anterior chamber may cause an acute and often transient elevation of IOP.

- The distinction between steroid responsiveness versus uveitic glaucoma may be achieved by changing treatment to a nonglaucomagenic anti-inflammatory agent (e.g., fluorometholone) or steroid-sparing systemic agents (e.g., methotrexate, anti–tumor necrosis factor [TNF] agents) without starting glaucoma drops.

- If the uveitis cannot be managed without continuing steroid therapy, then medical and, as needed, surgical glaucoma management are required.

Treatment and Prognosis

- The prognosis of uveitic glaucoma depends on the underlying disease and success of the treatment regimen.

- Treatment includes treating the underlying disease, ocular inflammation, and glaucoma.

- Systemic immunomodulatory medications may be necessary to provide control of the underlying disease. In patients with JIA, use of systemic anti-TNF agents is thought to lower the ocular complications of cataracts, band keratopathy, and glaucoma.

- Control of chronic uveitis, especially in JIA, may require chronic frequent topical steroids with slow weans over months to years.

- Mydriatic drops are essential in decreasing the risk of pupillary block by increasing the pupil size and breaking posterior synechiae.

- Elevated IOP is treated by determining the glaucoma mechanism (e.g., steroid-induced vs. iris bombe).

- Patients with glaucoma are treated primarily with topical antiglaucoma drops. A suggested general rule is that surgery is to be avoided when possible because the eyes often have an aggressive inflammatory response.

- Patients who do require surgery should be treated with preoperative oral prednisone as well as frequent topical prednisone.

- Goniotomy is an effective first-line surgical option for young patients with chronic uveitis and glaucoma without significant peripheral anterior synechia or iris bombe who fail medical glaucoma management.

- Trabeculectomy, especially in pediatric patients with uveitis, has a lower success rate because of aggressive scar formation.

- Glaucoma drainage devices are used in refractory cases and can provide good long-term glaucoma control comparable to those without uveitis.

- Intraocular lens implantation in children with uveitic cataracts may cause significant aggravation of the iritis and induce or worsen uveitis, which may cause or aggravate glaucoma.

REFERENCES

Freedman SF, Rodriguez-Rosa RE, Rojas MC, et al. Goniotomy for glaucoma secondary to chronic childhood uveitis. *Am J Ophthalmol.* 2002;133:617–621.

Rachmiel R, Trope GE, Buys YM, et al. Ahmed glaucoma valve implantation in uveitic glaucoma versus open-angle glaucoma patients. *Can J Ophthalmol.* 2008;43:462–467.

Sijssens KM, Rothova A, Berendschot TT, et al. Ocular hypertension and secondary glaucoma in children with uveitis. *Ophthalmology.* 2006;113:853. e2–859. e2.

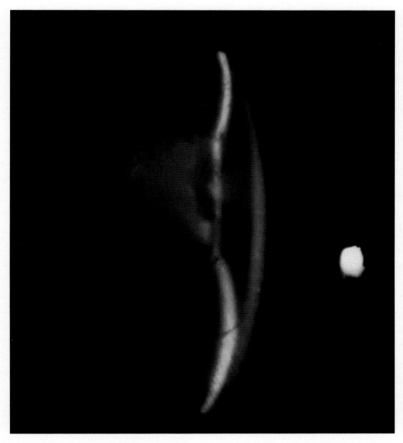

FIGURE 3-6. Uveitic glaucoma. Posterior synechia can result in pupillary block with iris bombe.

STURGE-WEBER SYNDROME

Encephalotrigeminal angiomatosis (Sturge-Weber syndrome) is a syndrome of port-wine birthmark—with or without ipsilateral risk of glaucoma—and central nervous system involvement, including possible developmental delay, seizures, and radiographic evidence of leptomeningeal calcification or cerebral atrophy. It is an example of *glaucoma associated with nonacquired systemic disease or syndrome.*

Epidemiology and Etiology

- There is no gender, race, or sexual predilection to the disorder.

- The classic Sturge-Weber port-wine birthmark respects the midline and follows the distribution of one or more of the trigeminal ganglion branches (Fig. 3-7).

- Up to 50% of patients develop glaucoma on the ipsilateral side, and eyes at higher risk have the upper eyelid affected.

- Whereas an onset of glaucoma early in life is thought to be the result of congenital goniodysgenesis, later-onset glaucoma, usually between 4 and 14 years, is related to elevated episcleral venous pressure.

- Sturge-Weber syndrome is caused by somatic mutation in the *GNAQ* gene.

- The risk for glaucoma is increased when choroidal hemangioma is present.

History

- The facial cutaneous lesion is usually the first component of Sturge-Weber syndrome to be observed and is visible at birth. It may become darker with age and is more noticeable in those with fair skin.

- Early-onset glaucoma presents with buphthalmos, epiphora, and photophobia as in primary congenital glaucoma.

- Later-onset glaucoma is diagnosed based on screening ophthalmic examination because there are usually no symptoms.

Signs

- The port-wine birthmark is a clinical marker to identify patients and eyes at risk for ocular complications.

- The hypervascularity of this disorder is evident on ocular examination with increased conjunctival and episcleral vascularity (Fig. 3-8) in up to 70% of patients.

- Heterochromia of the iris occurs in 10%, with increased pigment on the affected side caused by a relative increase in melanocyte activity or abnormal iris vasculature.

- Approximately 10% of patients with Sturge-Weber syndrome have bilateral disease.

- Diffuse choroidal hemangioma can be detected with indirect ophthalmoscopy showing indistinguishable choroidal markings (Fig. 3-9). It is usually seen in the posterior pole and can show thickening and elevation during adolescence and adulthood. Secondary changes to the overlying retina include vascular tortuosity, exudate, cystic changes, gliosis, and edema.

- On gonioscopy, blood visualized in Schlemm canal is suggestive of elevated episcleral venous pressure.

Differential Diagnosis

- Capillary hemangioma

- Klippel-Trenaunay-Weber syndrome (Sturge-Weber syndrome plus hemihypertrophy of soft and bony tissues)

- Transient nevus flammeus of infancy

- Primary congenital glaucoma

- JOAG

- Cutis marmorata telangiectasia congenita

- Phakomatosis pigmentovascularis

Diagnostic Evaluation

- Patients with a port-wine birthmark of the face involving any portion of the eyelids require referral for a complete ophthalmic evaluation with screening for glaucoma.

● Ocular testing for glaucoma includes a careful assessment of IOP, corneal diameter, corneal pachymetry (often elevated in those with Sturge-Weber syndrome), gonioscopy, cycloplegic refraction, axial length, and optic nerve cupping evaluation.

● Ocular ultrasonography may be useful, showing high internal reflectivity in a solid echogenic mass characteristic of choroidal hemangiomas and/or subretinal fluid. Enhanced depth OCT is also useful.

● Computed tomography scan and magnetic resonance imaging can be used to detect malformations in the brain and meninges.

Treatment and Prognosis

● Topical antiglaucoma medications are the initial treatment modality except in infancy when the treatment paradigm is usually surgical (goniotomy or trabeculotomy) as for primary congenital glaucoma.

● As the underlying pathophysiology becomes elevated episcleral venous pressure, medical treatment is still the desired first-line option, but trabeculectomy or drainage tube surgery may be needed.

● There is an increased risk of choroidal effusion and hemorrhage secondary to surgery.

● A diffuse choroidal hemangioma is associated with an increased risk of nonrhegmatogenous retinal detachment as well as vision loss caused by cystoid macular edema.

REFERENCES

Aggarwal NK, Gandham SB, Weinstein R, et al. Heterochromia iridis and pertinent clinical findings in patients with glaucoma associated with Sturge-Weber syndrome. *J Pediatr Ophthalmol Strabismus.* 2010;47:361–365.

Comi A, Levin AV, Kaplan E, et al. Leveraging a Sturge-Weber gene discovery: an agenda for future research. *Pediatric Neurology.* 2016;58:12–24.

Khaier A, Nischal KK, Espinosa M, Manoj B. Periocular port wine stain: the Great Ormond Street Hospital experience. *Ophthalmology.* 2011;118:2274–2278.

Maslin JS, Dorairaj SK, Ritch R. Sturge-Weber syndrome (encephalotrigeminal angiomatosis): recent advances and future challenges. *Asia Pac J Ophthalmol.* 2014;3:361–367.

Shiau T, Armogan N, Yan DB, Thomson HG, Levin AV. The role of episcleral venous pressure in glaucoma associated with Sturge-Weber syndrome. *J AAPOS.* 2012;16:61–64.

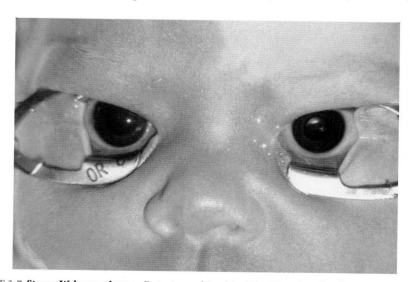

FIGURE 3-7. Sturge-Weber syndrome. Port-wine mark involving V1 to V3 on the right side and V2 to V3 on the left. The right eye has buphthalmos with corneal clouding.

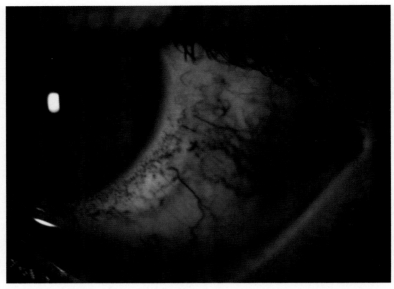

FIGURE 3-8. Sturge-Weber syndrome. Dilated tortuous conjunctival and episcleral vessels, ipsilateral to the side with port-wine mark (*not shown*).

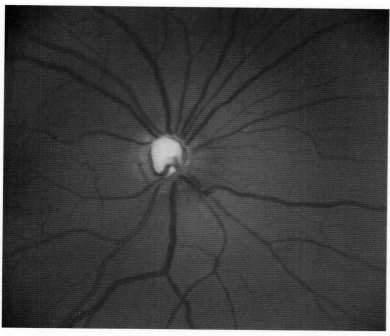

FIGURE 3-9. Choroidal hemangioma. Note the absence of choroidal markings and diffuse red-orange hue. Note the increased cup-to-disc ratio caused by glaucoma and the choroidal hemangioma.

CONGENITAL ECTROPION UVEAE

Congenital ectropion uveae is a rare disorder characterized by persistent cells of neural crest origin on the anterior surface of the iris and trabecular meshwork associated with varying degrees of ectropion uveae. Patients have an anterior insertion of the iris and dysgenesis of the anterior segment angle with an increased risk of glaucoma. It is an example of *glaucoma associated with nonacquired ocular anomalies.*

Epidemiology and Etiology

● Congenital ectropion uveae is a rare condition with an undefined incidence. It is almost always a unilateral disorder.

● Histopathologic studies have also described a fibrovascular surface membrane covering the anterior iris surface, suggesting that contraction causes the ectropion uveae and further growth into the angle inducing glaucoma.

● No genetic etiology or heritability has been described.

History

● Patients are usually asymptomatic and come to attention with concern about the iris/pupil appearance being different than the unaffected eye. Sometimes, the disorder is noted as an incidental finding during routine pediatric or ophthalmic examination.

Signs

● Slit-lamp biomicroscopy reveals iris posterior pigmented epithelium on the anterior surface of the iris (**Fig. 3-10**). The remainder of the iris appears smooth and cryptless with an overlying whitish coating.

● On gonioscopy, there is anterior insertion of the iris onto the trabecular meshwork and goniodysgenesis.

● IOP elevation and optic nerve cupping are indicative of the development of glaucoma.

● Mild ptosis with good levator function is reported in up to 50% of cases.

Differential Diagnosis

● Axenfeld-Rieger spectrum
● Anisocoria
● Iridocorneal endothelial syndrome
● Uveitis
● Rubeosis
● Trauma

Diagnostic Evaluation

● Congenital ectropion uveae can be associated with other anterior segment anomalies; thus, a thorough ophthalmoscopic and systemic evaluation is indicated.

● Reported rare associations include neurofibromatosis, facial hemihypertrophy, Axenfeld-Rieger spectrum, and Prader-Willi syndrome.

Treatment and Prognosis

● Although ectropion uveae is considered nonprogressive, this disorder is an indication for screening and continued surveillance for the development of glaucoma.

● Glaucoma almost inevitably develops, with the age of onset ranging from early childhood to adulthood.

● Treatment with standard antiglaucoma medications can result in an initial IOP-lowering effect but is short lived, and definitive treatment with trabeculectomy or glaucoma tube surgery is often required.

REFERENCES

Dowling JL Jr, Albert DM, Nelson LB, et al. Primary glaucoma associated with iridotrabecular dysgenesis and ectropion uveae. *Ophthalmology.* 1985;92:912–921.

Harasymowycz PJ, Papamatheakis DG, Eagle RC Jr, et al. Congenital ectropion uveae and glaucoma. *Arch Ophthalmol.* 2006;124:271–273.

Ritch R, Forbes M, Hetherington J Jr, et al. Congenital ectropion uveae with glaucoma. *Ophthalmology.* 1984;91:326–331.

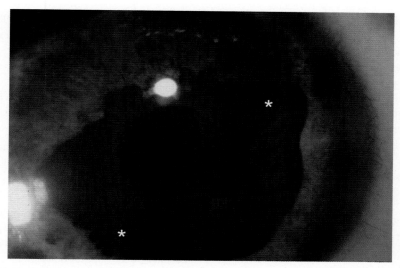

FIGURE 3-10. Congenital ectropion uveae. Iris pigment epithelium on the anterior surface of the iris (*asterisk*). Much of the remaining iris appears whitened with a loss of iris crypts.

ANIRIDIA

Aniridia is a panocular disorder with a cardinal feature of complete or partial iris absence with associated foveal hypoplasia, resulting in decreased visual acuity and early-onset nystagmus. Aniridia occurs as a result of a sporadic or autosomal dominant inherited mutation affecting the PAX6 gene, or deletion of nearby chromosomal material. It is an example of *glaucoma associated with nonacquired ocular anomalies.*

Epidemiology and Etiology

- The incidence of aniridia is 1 in 40,000 to 100,000.
- The amount of residual iris may differ between the two eyes.
- Disease-causing mutations have been reported in the PAX6 gene (11p13) or the allelic regulatory regions controlling its expression. The PAX6 gene encodes a transcriptional regulator that controls the expression of other genes involved in oculogenesis.
- Up to 20% of sporadic cases of aniridia have been found to have a deletion in 11p13 on cytogenetic testing. This deletion may involve the Wilms tumor gene (WT1) and intervening genes as part of WAGR syndrome (Wilms tumor, Aniridia, Genital anomalies, and Retardation).
- Patients with aniridia have up to a 50% lifetime risk of developing glaucoma.
- Glaucoma may be due to goniodysgenesis, hypoplasia/aplasia of Schlemm canal, or a closed angle due to migration anteriorly of the residual iris stub.

History

- Aniridia is discovered early in life usually by the presence of nystagmus in infancy.
- Visual acuity, when able to be tested, is often in the range of 20/100 to 20/200 but may be as good as 20/40 in patients with low expression.

- Patients may also experience photophobia.
- Only 20% of affected patients have a positive family history.

Signs

- Aniridia shows variable expression regarding the extent of iris abnormality and other ocular findings.
- Foveal hypoplasia is the primary cause of the decreased vision and is evident on ophthalmoscopy and can be confirmed with OCT.
- Other frequent ocular abnormalities include corneal pannus due to limbal stem cell deficiency, optic nerve hypoplasia, cataract (most commonly anterior pyramidal), and glaucoma.
- Less commonly, patients may have ectopia lentis, microphthalmia, ptosis, or Peters anomaly.
- Patients with aniridia and new-onset eye irritation require urgent evaluation for glaucoma as well as keratopathy.

Differential Diagnosis

- Axenfeld-Rieger spectrum
- Iris coloboma
- Gillespie syndrome
- Trauma or iatrogenic iris defect
- Bilateral congenital mydriasis
- Pharmacologic mydriasis

Diagnostic Evaluation

- Slit-lamp biomicroscopy is needed to detect corneal pannus, which often begins as peripheral gray superficial avascular changes.
- Examination under anesthesia is useful in obtaining complete ophthalmic testing, including IOP measurement and gonioscopy in young infants. In young children, the development and progression of glaucoma can be assessed by an increase in corneal diameter,

increase in the axial length, and loss of hyperopia or increased myopia on cycloplegic refraction.

- Gonioscopic examination reveals a rudimentary iris stub, rather than complete absence, possibly with areas of upturned iris blocking the trabecular meshwork (**Fig. 3-11**).

- In infants with significant corneal opacities, an anterior segment ultrasound biomicroscopy can demonstrate iris hypoplasia and show angle anomalies.

- Systemic findings associated with WAGR includes cryptorchidism and other genitourinary abnormalities, intellectual disability, neurologic abnormalities (e.g., hypertonia, hypotonia, epilepsy), skeletal anomalies (craniofacial anomalies, growth retardation, or scoliosis), hearing loss, and obesity.

Treatment and Prognosis

- Individuals without a family history of aniridia should undergo cytogenetic and molecular genetic testing to detect possible WAGR syndrome. Those with aniridia and *WT1* deletion require renal ultrasound every 3 months until approximately 8 years of age. In the absence of molecular testing to exclude WAGR, renal screening should be conducted every 4 to 6 months. Those without WAGR still require continued periodic ophthalmic examinations for glaucoma, corneal abnormalities, and cataracts.

- The treatment of glaucoma in aniridia is based on gonioscopy and age. Goniosurgery may be useful as a primary procedure, particularly in infants.

- The decision to perform cataract surgery requires consideration of other causes of diminished vision such as foveal hypoplasia, optic nerve hypoplasia, and nystagmus. Aniridic eyes can have poor zonular stability, affecting how the surgery is done and the type of lens implant used.

REFERENCES

Fischbach BV, Trout KL, Lewis J, et al. WAGR syndrome: a clinical review of 54 cases. *Pediatrics.* 2005;116:984–988.

Netland PA, Scott ML, Boyle JW, Lauderdale JD. Ocular and systemic findings in a survey of aniridia subjects. *J AAPOS.* 2011;5:562–566.

Ramaesh K, Ramaesh T, Dutton GN, et al. Evolving concepts on the pathogenic mechanisms of aniridia related keratopathy. *Int J Biochem Cell Biol.* 2005;37:547–557.

Schneider S, Osher RH, Burk SE, et al. Thinning of the anterior capsule associated with congenital aniridia. *J Cataract Refract Surg.* 2003;29:523–525.

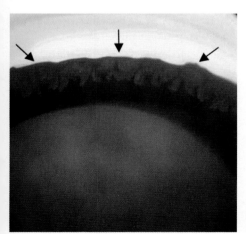

FIGURE 3-11. Aniridia. Gonioscopic view of aniridic eye with the iris root turned up in multiple places (*arrows*), obstructing the trabecular meshwork.

POSTERIOR EMBRYOTOXON

Posterior embryotoxon is the anterior displacement of Schwalbe's line and structurally represents an anteriorized junction of the peripheral termination of Descemet's membrane. Clinically, it appears as a white circumferential line on the inner surface of the cornea near the limbus. Histologically, it consists of collagen fibers covered by a thin layer of Descemet's membrane and endothelium.

Epidemiology and Etiology

• The prevalence of posterior embryotoxon is 6.8% to 32% of the general population. It may occur as an isolated finding or be associated with other anterior segment or systemic findings as in Axenfeld-Rieger spectrum and Alagille syndrome. It is considered a developmental neurocristopathy.

• There has not been a specific mutated gene associated with isolated posterior embryotoxon, but mutations in *PITX2*, *FOXC1*, and *JAG1* each are associated with the clinical findings of the syndromic forms.

• The risk of glaucoma in isolated posterior embryotoxon is not well defined but likely elevated. In Axenfeld-Rieger spectrum, the risk may be as high as 50%.

History

• Patients are usually asymptomatic. Often the disorder is noted as an incidental finding during slit-lamp biomicroscopy and gonioscopy.

Signs

• Posterior embryotoxon is visible with slit-lamp biomicroscopy as a fine silver-white circumferential line on the inner aspect of the cornea, anterior to the limbus (Fig. 3-12). It occurs more commonly nasally and temporally.

• The presence of iridocorneal strands to the posterior embryotoxon identifies the mildest form of Axenfeld-Rieger spectrum. With Axenfeld-Rieger spectrum, systemic anomalies include redundant periumbilical skin, abnormal facies, sensorineural hearing loss, skeletal malformations, and dental malformations.

• Ophthalmoscopic findings suggestive of Alagille syndrome include retinal pigment epithelial irregularities and optic nerve anomalies. It is a disorder primarily of biliary atresia or milder liver dysfunction and a characteristic facies.

Differential Diagnosis

• Axenfeld-Rieger spectrum

• Alagille syndrome

• Peters anomaly

• Cornea plana

• Anterior segment mesodermal dysgenesis

• Peripheral anterior synechiae

• Trauma

Diagnostic Evaluation

• The characteristic appearance of posterior embryotoxon should enable the clinician to make the diagnosis and differentiate it from other lesions. Gonioscopy can be used to identify cases that are not otherwise evident on slit-lamp examination.

• Although not needed to make the diagnosis, anterior segment OCT can also show the abnormality.

• Patients should have a complete ophthalmic examination, including IOP and dilated fundus examination. More aggressive monitoring is needed in patients with findings of Axenfeld-Rieger spectrum.

• Screening of family members may be helpful clinically because presentation is variable.

Treatment and Prognosis

- Medical management is the first line to treat glaucoma in this condition.

- Goniotomy and trabeculotomy when glaucoma is present are technically challenging and have lower success rates.

REFERENCES

Ozeki H, Shirai S, Majima A, et al. Clinical evaluation of posterior embryotoxon in one institution. *Jpn J Ophthalmol.* 1997;41:422–425.

Rennie CA, Chowdhury S, Khan J, et al. The prevalence and associated features of posterior embryotoxon in the general ophthalmic clinic. *Eye (Lond).* 2005;19:396–399.

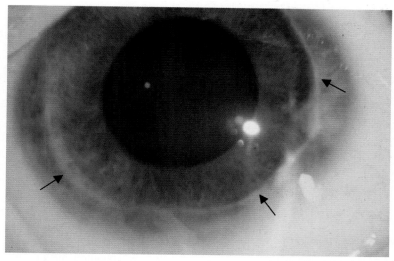

FIGURE 3-12. **Posterior embryotoxon** appears as a white or gray circumferential line anterior to the limbus (*arrows*).

CHAPTER

4

Iris Anomalies

Michael J. Bartiss and Bruce M. Schnall ■

CENTRAL PUPILLARY CYSTS (PUPILLARY MARGIN EPITHELIAL CYSTS)

Etiology

- Usually congenital in origin
- Can be acquired from cholinesterase-inhibiting eye drops, such as phospholine iodide, when used in young phakic patients to treat accommodative esotropia
- Rarely inherited

Symptoms

- Patients are usually asymptomatic.
- Pigmented epithelial cysts occurring at the pupillary border (Fig. 4-1)
- May be detected by a pediatrician on red reflex testing of neonate

Signs

- Pigmented cysts along the margin of the pupil of involved eyes
- Have a nontransparent lining (as opposed to iris stromal cysts)
- Rarely increase in size and typically remain stationary

Differential Diagnosis

- Iris stromal cysts
- Ciliary body cysts
- Iris melanoma

Treatment

- Congenital pupillary margin epithelial cysts rarely require treatment; they usually remain stationary in size or slowly involute over time.
- If size and location cause visual compromise, surgical intervention may be indicated.
- Acquired pupillary margin cysts from cholinesterase-inhibiting eye drops can be prevented with the use of phenylephrine (2.5%) eye drops daily.

Prognosis

- Excellent; rarely require treatment
- Complications can include formation of iris flocculi in cases of cyst rupture, glaucoma, and spontaneous intraocular detachment of the cysts.
- If treatment is required, can be treated with simple excision or yttrium aluminum garnet puncture

72

REFERENCES

Shields JA, Kline MW, Augsburger JJ. Primary iris cysts: a review of the literature and report of 62 cases. *Br J Ophthalmol.* 1984;68(3):152–166.

Shields JA, Shields CL, Lois N, et al. Iris cysts in children: classification, incidence and management: the 1998 Torrence A Makley, Jr., lecture. *Br J Ophthalmol.* 1999;83(3):334–338.

Sidoti PA, Valencia M, Chen M. Echographic evaluation of primary cysts of the iris pigment epithelium. *Am J Ophthalmol.* 1995;120:161–167.

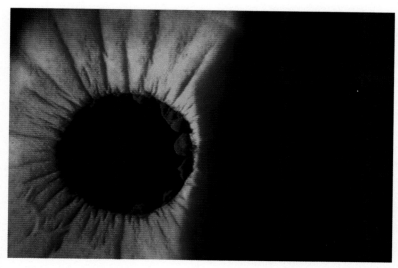

FIGURE 4-1. Pigmented epithelial cysts. Pigmented cysts along the margin of the pupil. (Courtesy of Judith Lavrich, MD.)

ANIRIDIA

Etiology

• Bilateral disorder characterized by underdevelopment (rather than true absence of the iris), with rudimentary iris located peripherally

• Associated with *PAX6* gene (control gene for eye morphogenesis) on chromosome 11p13, involving inability of single gene allele to activate transduction of developmental genes (haploinsufficiency)

• Often associated with foveal hypoplasia, nystagmus, glaucoma, optic nerve hypoplasia, cataracts, and acquired corneal pannus

• Autosomal dominant (complete penetrance with variable expressivity), autosomal recessive (Gillespie syndrome with mental retardation and cerebellar ataxia), and sporadic inheritance patterns

• Two-thirds of children with aniridia have affected parents.

• Sporadic aniridia is associated with an increased incidence of Wilms tumor.

• WAGR complex (Wilms tumor, aniridia, genitourinary malformations, and mental retardation) occurs from contiguous gene deletions.

Symptoms

• Clinical absence of the iris

• Subnormal visual acuity is common (usually less than 20/100).

• Nystagmus

• Photophobia

Signs

• Apparent bilateral absence or severe hypoplasia of iris (Fig. 4-2)

• Congenital nystagmus

• Acquired corneal pannus

• Strabismus

• Cataract

• Ectopia lentis

• Glaucoma

• Posterior synechiae

Differential Diagnosis

• Other causes of pupillary dilation (e.g., pharmacologically dilated pupils, Adie pupil)

Treatment

• Evaluation with a geneticist

• Screening for Wilms tumor includes abdominal ultrasonography evaluations every 3 months until 7 to 8 years of age.

• Screen for glaucoma and treat if present.

• Cataract surgery if visually significant cataract is present

• Maximize visual potential with appropriate refractive error correction.

• Polarized sun wear or use of Transitions spectacles lenses to decrease glare and photophobia

REFERENCES

Adeoti CO, Afolabi AA, Ashaye AO, et al. Bilateral sporadic aniridia: review of management. *Clin Ophthalmol.* 2010;4:1085–1089.

Lee H, Meyers K, Lanigan B, et al. Complications and visual prognosis in children with aniridia. *J Pediatr Ophthalmol Strabismus.* 2010;47(4):205–210.

Weissbart SB, Ayres BD. Management of aniridia and iris defects: an update on iris prosthesis options. *Curr Opin Ophthalmol.* 2016;27(3):244–249.

Yeung HH. Large Pupils in Infancy . . . Suspected Aniridia. Multisystemic smooth muscle dysfunction syndrome secondary to an ACTA2 mutation. *J Pediatr Ophthalmol Strabismus.* 2016;53(1):7, 8.

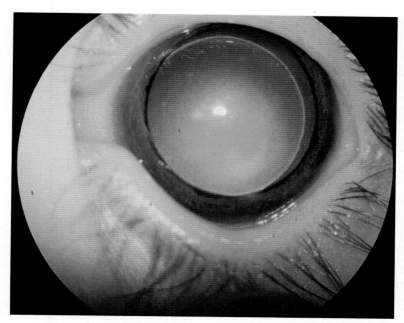

FIGURE 4-2. **Aniridia.** Severe hypoplasia of iris with outline of lens visible. (Courtesy of Alex V. Levin, MD, MHSc, Wills Eye Hospital, Philadelphia.)

BRUSHFIELD SPOTS

Etiology

- Occur in up to 90% of patients with Down syndrome (trisomy 21)
- Can be present in patients without Down syndrome

Symptoms

- Patients are asymptomatic.

Signs

- Whitish elevated spots on the anterior surface of the iris, often occurring in a concentric ring around the pupil (Fig. 4-3)
- Congenital, normal to hypercellular hypopigmented areas of iris tissue with surrounding relative stromal hypoplasia

Differential Diagnosis

- Wolfflin nodules (similar appearing nodules occurring in patients without Down syndrome, which are accumulations of fibrous tissue in the anterior border layer of the iris)
- Iris nevi
- Brushfield spots
- Juvenile xanthogranuloma (JXG)
- Iris mamillations

Treatment

- No treatment indicated

Prognosis

- No effect on visual function
- Severity of functional cognitive impairment of patients with trisomy 21 is extremely variable.

REFERENCES

Brooke Williams RD. Brushfield spots and Wolfflin nodules in the iris: an appraisal in handicapped children. *Dev Med Child Neurol.* 1981;23(5):646–649.

Ljubic A, Trajkovski V, Tesic M, Tojtovska B, Stankovic B. Ophthalmic manifestations in children and young adults with Down syndrome and congenital heart defects. *Ophthalmic Epidemiol.* 2015;22(2):123–129.

Shapiro BL. Down syndrome and associated congenital malformations [review]. *J Neural Transm Suppl.* 2003;(67):207–214.

Stirn Kranjc B. Ocular abnormalities and systemic disease in Down syndrome. *Strabismus.* 2012;20(2):74–77.

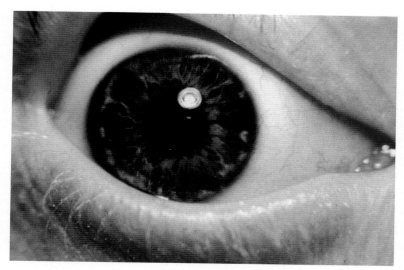

FIGURE 4-3. Brushfield spots. Hypopigmented elevated spots on the anterior iris surface in a concentric ring around the pupil. (Courtesy of Alex V. Levin, MD, MHSc, Wills Eye Hospital, Philadelphia.)

ECTOPIA LENTIS ET PUPILLAE

Etiology

- Autosomal recessive inherited, nonprogressive disorder in which the pupil and lens are displaced in opposite directions (pupil usually inferonasally and lens superotemporally)
- Posterior displacement of lens–iris diaphragm
- Typically bilateral and asymmetric
- Believed to occur during neuroectodermal tissue development (pigmented layers of iris, iris dilator, and zonules are all involved)

Symptoms

- Decreased uncorrected visual acuity secondary to dislocated lens

Signs

- Bilateral lens dislocation causing high myopia with astigmatism
- Asymmetrical, eccentrically located pupils (usually inferonasally)
- Slit-shaped or oval pupil (Fig. 4-4A)
- Persistent pupillary membrane is present in approximately 85% of affected individuals (Fig. 4-4B)
- Microspherophakia, miosis, and poor dilation with mydriatic agents
- Myopia, which may be severe
- May have an enlarged corneal diameter
- Cataract
- Abnormal iris transillumination
- Retinal detachment
- +/− Megalocornea

Differential Diagnosis

- Other causes for bilateral dislocated lenses, Marfan syndrome, homocystinuria, Weil-Marchesani syndrome, sulfite oxidase deficiency, hyperlysinemia
- Iris coloboma
- Trauma to iris sphincter
- After anterior segment surgery
- Corectopia
- Axenfeld-Rieger syndrome

Treatment

- Refractive error correction to maximize visual potential
- Anisometropic amblyopia often occurs in the more affected eye. Amblyopia should be treated with correction of refractive error and occlusion of the fellow eye.
- May develop a visually significant cataract and therefore may require cataract surgery
- Screen for glaucoma

Prognosis

- Nonprogressive; visual prognosis depends on timely treatment of refractive error. Amblyopia in more affected eye is often severe and may not respond to treatment.

REFERENCES

Byles DB, Nischal KK, Cheng H. Ectopia lentis et pupillae. A hypothesis revisited. *Ophthalmology.* 1998;105(7):1331–1336.

Colley A, Lloyd IC, Ridgway A, et al. Ectopia lentis et pupillae: the genetic aspects and differential diagnosis. *J Med Genet.* 1991;28(11):791–794.

Goldberg MF. Clinical manifestations of ectopia lentis et pupillae in 16 patients. *Ophthalmology.* 1988;95(8):1080–1087.

Sadiq MA, Vanderveen D. Genetics of ectopia lentis. *Semin Ophthalmol.* 2013;28(5–6):313–320.

Sharifi Y, Tjon-Fo-Sang MJ, Cruysberg JR, Maat-Kievit AJ. Ectopia lentis et pupillae in four generations caused by novel mutations in the *ADAMTSL4* gene. *Br J Ophthalmol.* 2013;97(5):583–587.

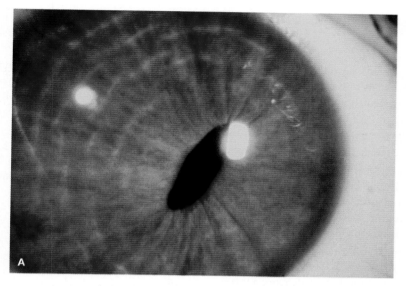

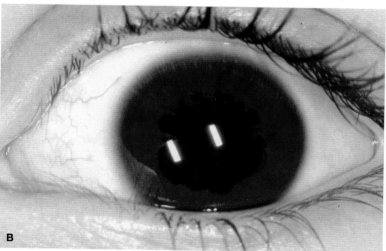

FIGURE 4-4. Ectopia lentis et pupillae. A. Inferonasally eccentrically located slit-shaped pupil. (Courtesy of Alex V. Levin, MD, MHSc, Wills Eye Hospital, Philadelphia.) **B.** Note the persistent pupillary membrane, which is being stretched in this pharmacologically dilated pupil. The superior edge of the dislocated lens is visible.

HETEROCHROMIA IRIDIS

Etiology

- A congenital or acquired condition characterized by a relative hyperpigmentation or hypopigmentation of the involved iris
- Acquired cases of hyperpigmented irides in children include trauma, siderosis, iris ectropion syndrome, chronic iridocyclitis, and extensive rubeosis as well as intraocular surgery and topical prostaglandin analog medications
- Ocular melanocytosis or oculodermal melanocytosis and sector iris hamartoma can also cause hyperpigmented irides.
- Congenital and acquired hypopigmented irides can occur because of Horner syndrome, Fuchs heterochromia, Waardenburg-Klein syndrome, nonpigmented iris tumors, and hypomelanosis of Ito.

Symptoms

- Patients are typically asymptomatic in the absence of rubeosis, increased intraocular pressure (IOP), and intraocular inflammation.

Signs

- Different-colored irides with or without anatomic iris abnormalities
- In cases of melanosis oculi, the more pigmented iris may appear thicker with mamillations (**Fig. 4-5**).
- Associated with miosis and ptosis (typically 2 mm) on the ipsilateral side in cases of Horner syndrome (**Fig. 4-6**)

Differential Diagnosis

- Differential diagnosis is extensive.
- Acquired cases of hyperpigmented irides in children include trauma, siderosis, iris ectropion syndrome, chronic iridocyclitis, and extensive rubeosis as well as intraocular surgery and topical prostaglandin analog medications.

- Ocular melanocytosis or oculodermal melanocytosis and sector iris hamartoma can also cause hyperpigmented irides.
- Congenital and acquired hypopigmented irides can occur because of Horner syndrome, Fuchs heterochromia, Waardenburg-Klein syndrome, nonpigmented iris tumors, and hypomelanosis of Ito.
- Neuroblastoma (located along the sympathetic chain) must be ruled out in cases of Horner syndrome, especially in acquired cases in children.

Treatment

- Assessment as to which iris has the abnormal color can often be assisted by assessing skin pigmentation, parental eye color, and earlier photographs of the patient.
- Timely and appropriate workup of acquired Horner syndrome
- Hearing testing if Waardenburg syndrome is suspected
- In cases of acquired hyperpigmentation, imaging may be needed to rule out an intraocular foreign body (siderosis) and intraocular tumor.

Prognosis

- Depends on the underlying cause

REFERENCES

Brazel SM, Sullivan TJ, Thorner PS, et al. Iris sector heterochromia as a marker for neural crest disease. *Arch Ophthalmol.* 1992;110(2):233–235.

Liu XZ, Newton VE, Read AP. Waardenburg syndrome type II: phenotypic findings and diagnostic criteria. *Am J Med Genet.* 1995;55(1):95–100.

Milunsky JM. Waardenburg syndrome type I. In: Pagon RA, Bird TC, Dolan CR, Stephens K, eds. *GeneReviews.* Seattle: University of Washington; 2004.

Radke P, Schimmenti LA, Schoonveld C, Bothun ED, Summers CG. The unique association of iris heterochromia with Hermansky-Pudlak syndrome. *J AAPOS.* 2013;17(5):542–544.

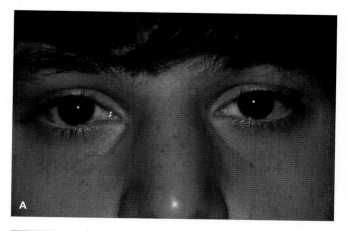

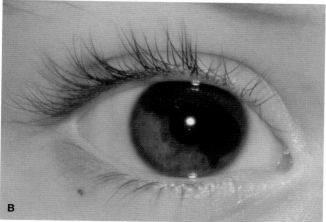

FIGURE 4-5. Heterochromia iridis. A. Right iris is more heavily pigmented in this child with melanosis oculi. **B.** Sector melanosis oculi.

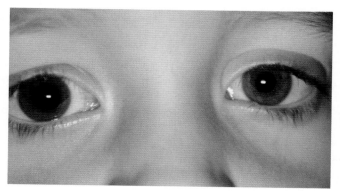

FIGURE 4-6. Left congenital Horner syndrome. Note the miotic pupil, mild ptosis, and hypopigmented iris on the left. The ptosis is best observed by looking at the distance from the corneal light reflex to the pupillary margin.

IRIS COLOBOMA

Etiology

● Typically bilateral inferonasal defect in the iris caused by failure of embryonic fissure closure during the fifth gestation week

● May be part of a spectrum of anatomic developmental abnormalities including microphthalmia

● Autosomal dominant inheritance in approximately 20% of cases

● Atypical iris colobomas located other than inferonasally can occur and are probably caused by developmental abnormalities of the anterior hyaloids and papillary membrane systems and are not associated with posterior segment colobomas

● Numerous chromosomal abnormalities, including trisomy 13, 4p-, 11q-13r, and 18r, are associated with colobomas.

● Numerous syndromes are associated with uveal colobomas, most notably CHARGE syndrome (coloboma of the eye or central nervous system anomalies, heart defects, atresia of the choanae, retardation of growth or development, genital or urinary defects, and ear anomalies or deafness).

● Other associated syndromes include Goltz syndrome (focal dermal hypoplasia), basal cell nevus syndrome, linear sebaceous syndrome, Klinefelter syndrome, and Goldenhar syndrome.

Symptoms

● Keyhole- or bulb-shaped pupil

● Patients are often asymptomatic if only the iris is involved.

● Patients are sometimes bothered by their cosmetic appearance.

● Visual acuity depends on involvement of the posterior segment.

Signs

● Inferonasal, lightbulb-shaped iris defect (Fig. 4-7)

● Colobomatous defect can also involve ciliary body, retina, choroid, and optic nerve. Lens zonules may be missing in a sector of the coloboma.

● Involvement may be asymmetric.

● Nystagmus presents in cases with concomitant bilateral optic nerve or macula involvement.

Differential Diagnosis

● Traumatic iris injury

● After an iridectomy

● Ectopic pupil

● Corectopia

Treatment

● Evaluation by a geneticist if other congenital anomalies are found or a syndrome is suspected

● Maximize visual acuity with appropriate refractive error correction.

● Colored contact lenses (with iris detail) are often helpful if psychosocial issues are present, especially in patients with lightly colored irides.

● Impact-resistant spectacles, especially in cases with functional vision in only one eye

Prognosis

● Visual prognosis depends on involvement of the optic disc and macula. Visual potential is very difficult to predict on the basis of clinical examination alone even in cases with significant posterior segment involvement.

● Visual acuity often remains stable after it has been maximized.

● Risk of retinal detachment

REFERENCES

Deml B, Reis LM, Lemyre E, Clark RD, Kariminejad A, Semina EV. Novel mutations in PAX6, OTX2 and NDP in anophthalmia, microphthalmia and coloboma. *Eur J Hum Genet.* 2016;24(4):535–541.

Mets MB, Erzurum SA. Uveal tract in infants. In: Isenberg SJ, ed. *The Eye in Infancy.* 2nd ed. St. Louis, MO: Mosby; 1994:308–317.

Onwochei BC, Simon JW, Bateman JB, et al. Ocular colobomata. *Surv Ophthalmol.* 2000;45:175–194.

Takkar B, Chandra P, Kumar V, Agrawal R. A case of iridofundal coloboma with persistent fetal vasculature and lens subluxation. *J AAPOS.* 2016;20(2):180–182.

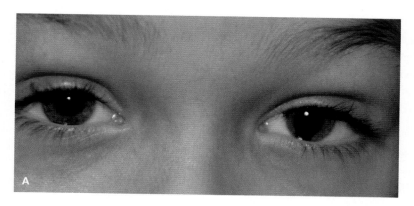

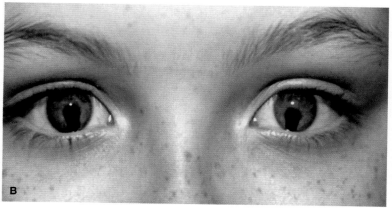

FIGURE 4-7. Iris coloboma. A. Unilateral iris coloboma. Lightbulb-shaped inferonasal defect in iris of the left eye. **B.** Bilateral iris coloboma.

IRIS STROMAL CYSTS

Etiology

• Probably occur because of sequestration of epithelial cells during embryologic development

• Typically contain goblet cells

Symptoms

• Can enlarge over time, obstructing the visual axis and causing decreased visual acuity

• Iritis with increased IOP and photophobia can occur if cysts leak.

• Often diagnosed during infancy

Signs

• Clear to whitish appearing cyst on the anterior surface of the iris (**Fig. 4-8**)

• Epithelium-lined cysts occurring on the anterior surface of the iris with a visible vasculature

• May enlarge, causing decreased vision by obstructing the visual axis, iritis (from cyst leakage), corneal decompensation, and glaucoma

Differential Diagnosis

• Secondary cyst formation from traumatic or surgical epithelial implantation

• Solid iris tumors

• Ciliary body tumors

Treatment

• Surgical excision with sector iridectomy may be the preferred treatment because it may lessen risk of cyst leakage causing iritis and increased IOP and will better the chance of removing the entire tumor, lessening the chance of recurrence.

Prognosis

• Guarded

REFERENCES

Casey M, Cohen KL, Wallace DK. Recurrence of iris stromal cyst following aspiration and resection. *J AAPOS.* 2002;6(4):255–256.

Pochop P, Mahelková G, Cendelín J, Petrušková D. Early detection of recurrent primary iris stromal cyst using ultrasound biomicroscopy. *J AAPOS.* 2014;18(2):184–186.

Shields CL, Arepalli S, Lally EB, Lally SE, Shields JA. Iris stromal cyst management with absolute alcohol-induced sclerosis in 16 patients. *JAMA Ophthalmol.* 2014;132(6):703–708.

Shields JA, Shields CL, Lois N, Mercado G. Iris cysts in children: classification, incidence and management: the 1998 Torrence A Makley, Jr., lecture. *Br J Ophthalmol.* 1999;83(3):334–338.

Shields JA. Primary cysts of the iris. *Trans Am Ophthalmol Soc.* 1981;79:771–809.

Wiwatwongwana A, Ittipunkul N, Wiwatwongwana D. Ab externo laser photocoagulation for the treatment of spontaneous iris stromal cyst. *Graefes Arch Clin Exp Ophthalmol.* 2012;250(1):155–156.

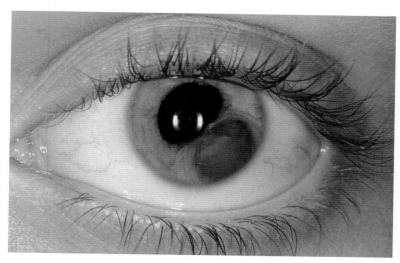

FIGURE 4-8. **Iris stromal cyst.** Whitish clear-appearing cyst in iris stroma. (Courtesy of Jerry Shields, MD.)

JUVENILE XANTHOGRANULOMA

Etiology

- Disorder of unknown etiology characterized by abnormal proliferation of non-Langerhans histiocytes with Touton giant cells occurring predominantly in infancy and early childhood
- Most often occurs unilaterally
- Common in children with neurofibromatosis type 1 (NF1)
- Optic nerve, retina, and choroid can also be infiltrated

Symptoms

- May cause spontaneous hyphema with decreased vision and increased IOP, corneal enlargement, and perilimbal flush and photophobia
- Children with skin lesions of JXG are routinely screened for eye involvement.

Signs

- Can present as vascular, discrete reddish or yellow lesions or diffusely causing heterochromia irides (Fig. 4-9)
- Spontaneous or recurrent unilateral hyphema
- Skin lesions appear as an acquired tan or orange papule or nodule. Skin lesions are self-limited.

Differential Diagnosis

- Leukemic infiltrates
- Lisch nodules
- Brushfield spots
- Iris mamillations

Treatment

- Biopsy of skin lesion to confirm diagnosis in patients with concomitant skin lesions
- Anterior chamber paracentesis can be performed in patients without skin lesions.
- Avoid iris biopsy because of the high risk of hemorrhage.
- Topical or subconjunctival steroids can be used as the first line of treatment.
- Radiotherapy (with dose not exceeding 500 cGy) can be used if the initial treatment is unsuccessful and the risk-to-benefit ratio is acceptable.

Prognosis

- Good with timely and appropriate diagnosis and treatment

REFERENCES

DeBarge LR, Chan CC, Greenberg SC, et al. Chorioretinal, iris, and ciliary body infiltration by juvenile xanthogranuloma masquerading as uveitis. *Surv Ophthalmol.* 1994;39(1):65–71.

Kontos G, Borooah S, Khan A, Fleck BW, Coupland SE. The epidemiology, clinical characteristics, histopathology and management of juvenile- and adult-onset corneoscleral limbus xanthogranuloma. *Graefes Arch Clin Exp Ophthalmol.* 2016;254(3):413–420.

Samara WA, Khoo CT, Say EA, et al. Juvenile xanthogranuloma involving the eye and ocular adnexa: tumor control, visual outcomes, and globe salvage in 30 patients. *Ophthalmology.* 2015;122(10):2130–2138.

Shields CL, Shields JA, Buchanon HW. Solitary orbital involvement with juvenile xanthogranuloma. *Arch Ophthalmol.* 1990;108(11):1587–1589.

Surapaneni KR, Wang AL, Burkat CN. Juvenile xanthogranuloma. *Ophthalmology.* 2015;122(5):870.

Zamir E, Wang RC, Krishnakumar S, et al. Juvenile xanthogranuloma masquerading as pediatric chronic uveitis: a clinicopathologic study. *Surv Ophthalmol.* 2001;46(2):164–171.

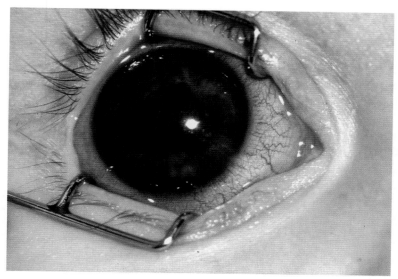

FIGURE 4-9. JXG. Reddish-yellow lesions on iris with signs of past intraocular inflammation. (Courtesy of Alex V. Levin, MD, MHSc, Wills Eye Hospital, Philadelphia.)

LISCH NODULES

Etiology

- Discrete dome-shaped nodules, which are melanocytic hamartomas occurring in patients with NF1

- Occurs in children affected with NF1 at an incidence approximately equal to 10 times the child's age in years up to age 9

- Rare in NF2

Symptoms

- Nodules do not affect vision directly.

Signs

- Bilaterally occurring, discrete dome-shaped nodules appearing anywhere on the anterior iris surface (including the angle when gonioscopic observation may be necessary to see them) (Fig. 4-10)

- Most are round, mildly pigmented (tan), and may be distributed more on the inferior iris surface than the superior iris surface.

- NF1 sometimes associated with pulsatile exophthalmos secondary to absence of the greater wing of the sphenoid bone and plexiform neuroma of the eyelid, giving an S-shaped deformity to the upper eyelid in early childhood

Differential Diagnosis

- Iris nevi
- Brushfield spots
- JXG
- Iris mamillations

Treatment

- Observation of Lisch nodules in a child not carrying the diagnosis of NF should trigger a workup for the disease and evaluation of family members.

Prognosis

- Depends on the presence or absence of concomitant abnormalities associated with NF, such as optic nerve glioma

REFERENCES

Friedman JM. Neurofibromatosis 1. In: Pagon RA, Bird TC, Dolan CR, Stephens K, eds. *GeneReviews*. Seattle: University of Washington; 2009.

Jett K, Friedman JM. Clinical and genetic aspects of neurofibromatosis 1 [review]. *Genet Med.* 2010;12(1):1–11.

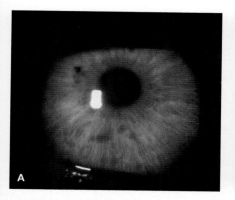

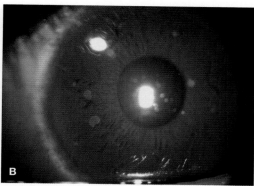

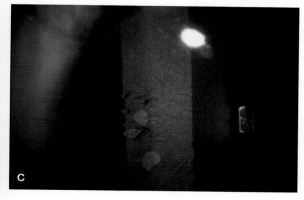

FIGURE 4-10. Lisch nodules. Discrete, mildly pigmented dome-shaped nodules on the anterior iris surface of a white patient (**A**) and an African American patient (**B**). **C.** Slit-lamp photo of Lisch nodules on the anterior iris surface of an African American patient.

MELANOSIS OCULI (OCULAR MELANOCYTOSIS)

Etiology

• Congenital

• Increase in the number of melanocytes in the iris, sclera, uvea, and surrounding tissues. The melanocytes are located deep within the sclera, yielding a slate-gray pigmentation rather than the normal brownish pigmentation usually associated with melanin.

Symptoms

• Increased pigmentation of the iris; discoloration of the sclera

• Usually none unless associated with increased IOP or malignant melanoma

Signs

• A congenital, flat, slate-gray discoloration of the sclera, iris, and uveal tract (Fig. 4-11). The conjunctiva is not involved.

• Most often unilateral but can occur bilaterally

• Eyelid skin may be involved as well. Some patients, especially those of Asian ancestry, may have associated increased pigmentation of the eyelid and adjacent skin (oculodermal melanocytosis, nevus of Ota), which can appear brown, bluish, or black without another skin abnormality (Fig. 4-12).

Differential Diagnosis

• Bilateral patches of slate-gray scleral pigmentation common in Asian and African American children (which have no clinical significance)

• Congenital nevocellular nevus of the eyelids

• Conjunctival nevi

• Melanosis of the sclera and skin sometimes associated with Sturge-Weber syndrome and Klippel-Trenaunay-Weber syndrome

Treatment

• Increased risk of glaucoma and malignant melanoma occurs with increased intraocular pigmentation.

• Routine screening for glaucoma and dilated fundus examination yearly to rule out uveal melanoma

Prognosis

• Depends on the presence or absence of glaucoma and malignant melanoma

REFERENCES

Chernoff KA, Schaffer JV, Cutaneous and ocular manifestations of neurocutaneous syndromes. *Clin Dermatol.* 2016;34(2):183–204.

Daitch Z, Shields CL, Say EA, Mashayekhi A, Shields JA. Sub-millimeter choroidal melanoma detection by enhanced depth imaging optical coherence tomography in a patient with oculodermal melanocytosis. *Retin Cases Brief Rep.* 2016;10(1):6–10.

Ellis FD. Selected pigmented fundus lesions of children. *J AAPOS.* 2005;9(4):306–314.

Gray ME, Shaikh AH, Corrêa ZM, Augsburger JJ. Primary uveal melanoma in a 4-year-old black child. *J AAPOS.* 2013;17(5):551–553.

Honavar SG, Shields CL, Singh AD, et al. Two discrete choroidal melanomas in an eye with ocular melanocytosis [review]. *Surv Ophthalmol.* 2002;47(1):36–41.

Mashayekhi A, Kaliki S, Walker B, et al. Metastasis from uveal melanoma associated with congenital ocular melanocytosis: amatched study. *Ophthalmology.* 2013;120(7):1465–1468.

Shields CL, Kaliki S, Livesey M, et al. Association of ocular and oculodermal melanocytosis with the rate of uveal melanoma metastasis: analysis of 7872 consecutive eyes. *JAMA Ophthalmol.* 2013;131(8):993–1003.

Shields CL, Nickerson SJ, Al-Dahmash S, Shields JA. Waardenburg syndrome: iris and choroidal hypopigmentation: findings on anterior and posterior segment imaging. *JAMA Ophthalmol.* 2013;131(9):1167–1173.

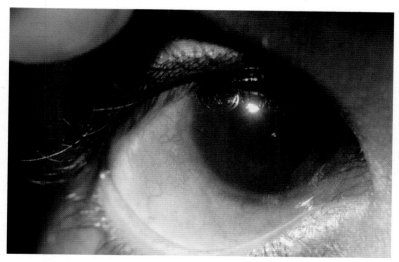

FIGURE 4-11. Ocular melanocytosis. Flat, slate-gray discoloration of sclera.

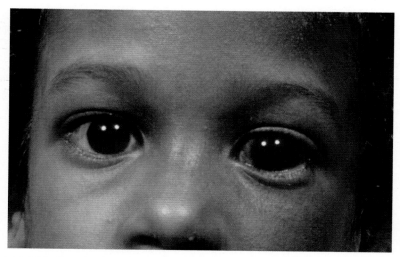

FIGURE 4-12. Oculodermal melanocytosis. Note the increased pigmentation of the sclera, eyelids, and adjacent skin on the left side.

PERSISTENT PUPILLARY MEMBRANE

Etiology

● Common developmental abnormality of the iris

● Results from incomplete involution of anterior tunic vasculosa lentis (which normally begins to involute at the beginning of the third trimester)

Symptoms

● Visually insignificant in almost all but most severely involved eyes

Signs

● Membranes attach to iris collarette, may be free floating, or span the pupil and attach on the opposite side to the iris or to the anterior lens surface (which may be extensive) (Fig. 4-13).

● Can be associated with cataract (usually centrally located), microcornea, megalocornea, microphthalmos, and coloboma

Differential Diagnosis

● Fibrinous anterior uveitis

● Ectopia lentis et pupillae

Treatment

● In the rare cases when vision is affected by persistent papillary membranes, medical therapy (papillary dilation and amblyopia therapy) is usually adequate.

● Surgical interventions (including iridectomy, removal of membrane, and laser therapy) have been attempted in the past with mixed success.

Prognosis

● Usually very good without treatment

REFERENCES

Kothari M, Mody K. Excision of persistent pupillary membrane using a suction cutter. *J Pediatr Ophthalmol Strabismus.* 2009;46(3):187.

Kurt E. A patient with bilateral persistent pupillary membrane: a conservative approach. *J Pediatr Ophthalmol Strabismus.* 2009;46(5):300–302.

Meyer-Rüsenberg B, Thill M, Vujancevic S, et al. Conservative management of bilateral persistent pupillary membranes with 18 years of follow-up. *Graefes Arch Clin Exp Ophthalmol.* 2010;248(7):1053–1054.

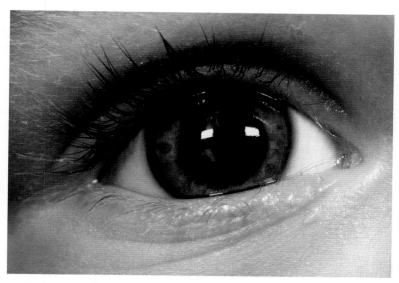

FIGURE 4-13. Persistent pupillary membrane spanning the pupil and attaching to the anterior lens surface. (Courtesy of Alex V. Levin, MD, MHSc, Wills Eye Hospital, Philadelphia.)

POSTERIOR SYNECHIAE

Etiology

● Congenital adhesions from the iris margin to the lens capsule. Congenital adhesions may occur in association with cataract, intrauterine inflammation, and aniridia. May also represent isolated remnants of the tunica vasculosa lentis (which are benign).

● Acquired adhesions occur more frequently and are most often associated with iridocyclitis.

Symptoms

● Patients are typically asymptomatic unless associated iridocyclitis or active sarcoidosis is present.

Signs

● Misshaped pupil

● Adhesions between the iris margin and lens capsule (Fig. 4-14)

● Congenital synechia may be associated with small anterior polar cataract at the point where the iris inserts into the lens capsule.

● Pigments on the anterior lens capsule surface often found in a circular pattern after intraocular inflammatory synechiae are broken.

Differential Diagnosis

● Persistent pupillary membrane

● Acquired synechia can also be associated with sarcoidosis, with Koeppe or Busacca nodules.

Treatment

● Congenital synechia with anterior polar cataract may be associated with hyperopia astigmatism and anisometropic amblyopia.

● Pharmacologic treatment with eye drops to dilate the pupil can often successfully break fresh acquired synechia.

● Surgical synechialysis is sometimes required when posterior synechia are present for a significant amount of the circumference of the papillary aperture or risk of angle closure is present.

REFERENCES

Kadayifçilar S, Eldem B, Tumer B. Uveitis in childhood. *J Pediatr Ophthalmol Strabismus.* 2003;40(6):335–340.
Levy-Clarke GA, Nussenblatt RB, Smith JA. Management of chronic pediatric uveitis [review]. *Curr Opin Ophthalmol.* 2005;16(5):281–288.

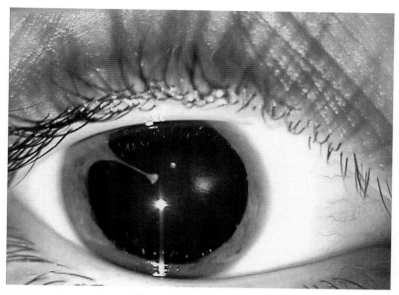

FIGURE 4-14. Posterior synechiae. Adhesion between iris and anterior lens surface. (Courtesy of Jonathan Salvin, MD.)

AXENFELD-RIEGER ANOMALY

Etiology

- Part of a group of anterior segment defects (formerly known as mesodermal dysgenesis) with both genotypic and phenotypic overlap

- Iris and pupil abnormalities associated with anterior displacement of Schwalbe line with iris bands extending to the cornea (Axenfeld anomaly)

- Autosomal dominant inheritance is most common.

- Called Rieger syndrome if associated with dental and skeletal abnormalities

- Mutations in *RIEG1/PITX2* gene (gene that regulates expansion of other genes during embryological development) on chromosome 4q25 have been identified.

- Mutations in *FOXC1* (transcription factor gene) also associated with this condition

Symptoms

- Abnormally shaped iris or pupil

- Photophobia secondary to significant iridodysgenesis

Signs

- Prominent iris processes that insert to an anteriorly displaced Schwalbe line (Fig. 4-15); may have a thinned iris stroma, bilateral iridodysgenesis with iris transillumination, peripheral anterior synechia, an eccentric and displaced pupil

Differential Diagnosis

- Posterior embryotoxon

- Peters anomaly

- Ectopic pupil

Treatment

- Fifty percent risk of glaucoma development; timely and appropriate monitoring for the development of glaucoma, including gonioscopy

- No treatment for underlying abnormalities

- Appropriate sunwear for photophobia symptoms

- Colored contact lens for glare and cosmesis concerns

- Genetic evaluation if systemic involvement is suspected

Prognosis

- Depends on involvement of the anterior segment and the presence of glaucoma

REFERENCES

Cella W, de Vasconcellos JP, de Melo MB, et al. Structural assessment of PITX2, FOXC1, CYP1B1, and GJA1 genes in patients with Axenfeld-Rieger syndrome with developmental glaucoma. *Invest Ophthalmol Vis Sci.* 2006;47(5):1803–1809.

Micheal S, Siddiqui SN, Zafar SN, et al. Whole exome sequencing identifies a heterozygous missense variant in the PRDM5 gene in a family with Axenfeld-Rieger syndrome. *Neurogenetics.* 2016;17(1):17–23.

Singh DV, Sharma YR, Azad RV, et al. Familial ectopia lentis with Axenfeld-Rieger anomaly. *J Pediatr Ophthalmol Strabismus.* 2007;44(1):59–61.

Yi K, Walden PG, Chen TC. What's your diagnosis? Axenfeld-Rieger anomaly without glaucoma. *J Pediatr Ophthalmol Strabismus.* 2007;44(6):333, 355.

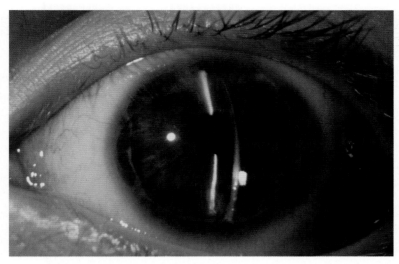

FIGURE 4-15. Axenfeld-Rieger anomaly. Iris processes inserting to an anteriorly displaced Schwalbe line. (Courtesy of Alex V. Levin, MD, MHSc, Wills Eye Hospital, Philadelphia.)

IRIS FLOCCULI

Etiology

- Arise from iris pigment epithelium (congenital)

Symptoms

- Rarely cause visual symptoms

Signs

- Spherical or teardrop-shaped lesions overlapping pupil (Fig. 4-16)

Differential Diagnosis

- Iris stromal cysts

Treatment

- Can be surgically removed

Prognosis

- Excellent visual prognosis

- Associated with gene mutation in *ACTA2* and/or *MYH11* gene (smooth muscle gene)

- These gene defects are associated with familial thoracic aortic aneurysm and dissection (TAAD) (Fig. 4-17).

- Long-term follow-up for TAAD is required as there is a reported case of TAAD occurring 55 years after diagnosis of iris flocculi.

REFERENCES

Shields JA, Magrath GN, Shields C, et al. Dissecting aortic aneurysm 55 years after diagnosis of iris floccule. *Ocul Oncol Pathol.* 2016;2(4):222–225.

Shields JA, Shields CL, Lois N, Mercado G. Iris cysts in childhood: classification, incidence, and management. *Br J Ophthalmol.* 1999;83:334–338.

Willoughby CE, McGimpsey SJ, McConnell V. Iris flocculi are an ocular marker of smooth muscle-actin (ACTA2) mutation in familial thoracic aortic aneurysms leading to acute aortic dissections (TAAD). *Investigative Ophthalmol Vis Sci.* 2008;9(13):3121.

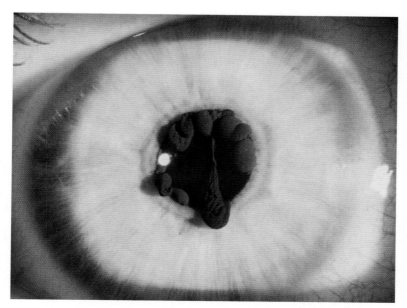

FIGURE 4-16. **Iris flocculi** overlapping pupil. (Courtesy of Jerry Shields, Wills Eye Hospital.)

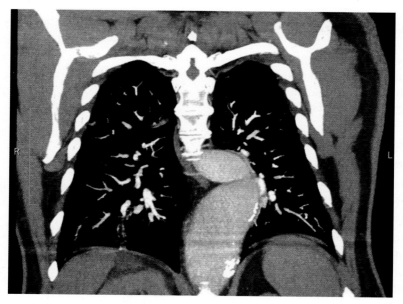

FIGURE 4-17. **Thoracic acute aneurysm and dissection**—TAAD. (Courtesy of Jerry Shields, Wills Eye Hospital.)

Lens Anomalies

Caroline DeBenedictis ■

CONGENITAL AND DEVELOPMENTAL CATARACTS

A cataract is an opacification of the lens inside the eye. Congenital cataracts are present at or soon after birth, whereas developmental cataracts develop during childhood. They can be unilateral or bilateral and cause obstruction of the visual axis. This leads to amblyopia, decreased visual acuity, or blindness (Fig. 5-1).

Etiology
- The prevalence is 1 to 4.24 per 10,000 children.
- Idiopathic (60% bilateral cases, 80% unilateral cases)
- Familial (30% cases)
- Most common morphologies: total cataract (31%), nuclear (27%), posterior subcapsular (27%)
- Genetic and metabolic diseases associated with cataract
  - Galactosemia
  - Alport syndrome
  - Fabry disease
  - Myotonic dystrophy
  - Diabetes mellitus
  - Trisomy 21
  - Trisomy 18
  - Trisomy 13
- Systemic illnesses associated with cataract include:
  - Juvenile idiopathic arthritis
  - Systemic lupus erythematosus
  - Malignancies
- Ocular abnormalities associated with cataract include:
  - Aniridia
  - Persistent hyperplastic primary vitreous
  - Anterior segment dysgenesis
- Maternal infection associated with cataract includes:
  - Rubella
  - Cytomegalovirus
  - Varicella
  - Herpes simplex virus
  - Toxoplasmosis
  - Syphilis

Signs and Symptoms

- Variable degree of lens opacification (small spots to total opacification)
- Variation of color changes (dark spots, white discoloration, total leukocoria)
- Decreased visual acuity
- Asymmetric, diminished, or absent red reflex
- Nystagmus
- Photophobia
- Strabismus
- Failure to meet developmental milestones
- Poor visual development in infants
- Poor visual function in older children

Diagnostic Evaluation

- Detailed history with specific attention to family history, trauma, systemic or topical steroid use, radiation exposure, maternal infection, systemic illness in child, and visual developmental milestones or visual changes
- Physical examination includes complete ophthalmologic examination with visual acuity testing, slit-lamp examination, pupillary dilation, retinoscopy, and indirect ophthalmoscopy
- B-scan ultrasonography
- Infants may require general anesthesia for full examination.
- Full physical examination with attention paid to growth and developmental milestones and appropriate referral for genetic, infectious, and metabolic testing

Treatment

- Visually significant cataract requires surgery with or without intraocular lens implant: cataract >3 mm, dense cataract, cataract preventing refraction, poor red reflex associated with nystagmus or strabismus
- Congenital visually significant cataracts require initiation of treatment within 4 to 8 weeks of life depending on laterality.
- Developmental cataracts in children younger than 7 years of age require initiation of treatment within weeks after diagnosis to avoid development or delay in treatment of amblyopia.
- Partial cataracts may require surgery or may be managed medically (glasses, patching, pupil dilation) depending on the extent of the cataract and surgical risks. If visual acuity can be accurately measured to be better than 20/50, medical management should be considered. If the visual acuity cannot be accurately measured or is measured to be 20/50 or worse, surgery should be considered.
- Postoperative aphakic refractive correction (glasses or contact lenses) initiated as soon as possible after surgery with appropriate treatment for amblyopia
- Appropriate referral of patient for evaluation and treatment of any underlying disease

Prognosis

- Depends on the age at diagnosis, morphology, laterality, concomitant ocular or systemic disease, and surgical complications
- In young children, postoperative prognosis depends on adherence to amblyopia treatment.

REFERENCES

Amaya L, Taylor D, Russell-Eggitt I, et al. The morphology and natural history of childhood cataracts. *Surv Ophthalmol.* 2003;48:125–144.

Lim Z, Rubab S, Chan YH, et al. Pediatric cataract: the Toronto experience-etiology. *Am J Ophthalmol.* 2010;149(6):887–892.

Lin AA, Buckley EG. Update on pediatric cataract surgery and intraocular lens implantation. *Curr Opin Ophthalmol.* 2010;21(1):55–59.

Wu X, Long E, Lin H, et al. Prevalence and epidemiological characteristics of congenital cataract: a systematic review and meta-analysis. *Sci Rep.* 2016;6:28564.

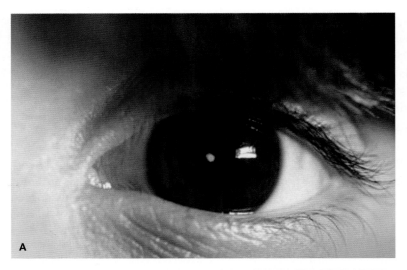

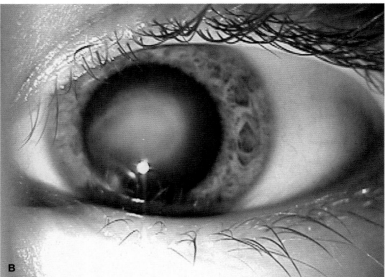

FIGURE 5-1. **Congenital cataract.** **A.** Anterior polar cataract: central anterior lens opacity generally less than 1 mm in diameter. These are rarely visually significant. **B.** Congenital nuclear cataract: large central nuclear opacity. This cataract is visually significant and requires surgical removal.

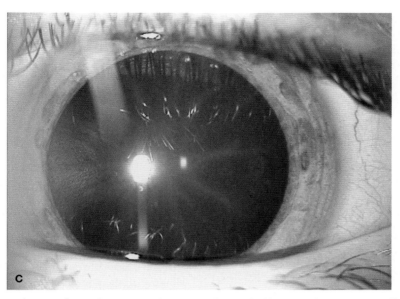

FIGURE 5-1. (*continued*) **C.** Stellate congenital cataract: stellate, spoke-like cortical lens opacity. Initially, this may not be visually significant, but it may progress to a total opacity.

ECTOPIA LENTIS

Ectopia lentis is the displacement of the lens of the eye (**Fig. 5-2**). Subluxation is defined as partial dislocation with the lens remaining attached to the ciliary body via the lens zonules. Luxation is the complete detachment of the lens from the ciliary body.

Etiology

- Trauma
- Congenital
- Ocular conditions
  - Simple ectopia lentis
  - Ectopia lentis et pupillae
  - Spherophakia/microspherophakia
  - Aniridia
  - Iris coloboma
  - Congenital glaucoma
  - Retinitis pigmentosa
  - Axenfeld-Rieger syndrome
  - Ciliary medulloepithelioma
  - Ciliary block glaucoma
- Systemic diseases associated with ectopia lentis:
  - Marfan syndrome
  - Homocystinuria
  - Weill-Marchesani syndrome
  - Ehlers-Danlos syndrome
  - Sulfite oxidase deficiency
  - Hyperlysinemia
  - Congenital syphilis
  - Crouzon syndrome
  - Apert disease
  - Myotonic dystrophy

Symptoms

- Mild to severely decreased visual acuity due to progressive or acute changes in refractive error
- Pain associated with pupillary block glaucoma

Signs

- Partial lens displacement posteriorly or anteriorly
- Complete lens displacement into anterior chamber or posterior pole
- Pupillary block glaucoma
- Induced irregular refractive errors (irregular astigmatism, high myopia, or aphakia)
- Amblyopia
- Iridodonesis

Diagnostic Evaluation

- Detailed history to determine the etiology with special attention paid to recent head, orbit, or eye trauma
- Full ocular exam including visual acuity, slit-lamp examination, and dilated fundoscopic examination
- Appropriate genetic, metabolic, and/or infectious studies if trauma is ruled out

Treatment

- Refractive correction with corrective lenses
- Amblyopia management
- Lensectomy with postoperative aphakic glasses or contact lenses
- Lensectomy with intraocular lens implantation if possible
- Treatment of secondary ocular conditions (i.e., pupillary block glaucoma)
- Refer to appropriate specialist for evaluation and treatment of underlying medical condition.

Prognosis

- Ninety percent of patients have a visual acuity of 20/40 or better after surgery with appropriate refractive correction.

REFERENCES

Colley A, Lloyd IC, Ridgway A, et al. Ectopia lentis et pupillae; the genetic aspects and differential diagnosis. *J Med Genet.* 1991;28(11):791–794.

Gupta NK, Simon JW, Walton DS, et al. Bilateral ectopia lentis as a presenting feature of medulloepithelioma. *JAAPOS.* 2001;5(4):255–257.

Neely DE, Plager DA. Management of ectopia lentis in children. *Ophthalmol Clin North Am.* 2001;14(3): 493–499.

Young TL. Ophthalmic genetics/inherited eye disease. *Curr Opin Ophthalmol.* 2003;14(5):296–303.

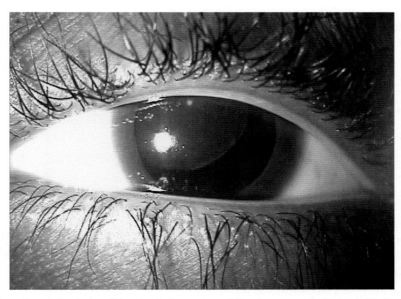

FIGURE 5-2. Ectopia lentis: lens dislocation in the superonasal direction more typically seen in Marfan syndrome.

ANTERIOR LENTICONUS

Anterior lenticonus is the anterior protrusion of the anterior lens through a weak or thin portion of the anterior lenticular capsule, often with associated lens opacification (Fig. 5-3).

Etiology

- May be associated with anterior subcapsular or anterior polar cataracts
- Alport syndrome, an inherited disorder (X-linked in 85%) with hemorrhagic nephritis and sensorineural hearing loss
- Trauma

Symptoms

- Small (<2–3 mm) may have no symptoms
- Blurred vision or induced amblyopia

Signs

- Typically bilateral
- Central, conical anterior protrusion of the anterior lens capsule seen on slit-lamp examination (Fig. 5-3)
- Central "oil-droplet" appearance on red reflex examination
- Induced myopic or astigmatic refractive errors
- Color changes such as whitened red reflex

Diagnosis

- Detailed history, including family history for Alport syndrome
- Complete eye examination, including visual acuity, slit-lamp examination, dilated fundoscopic examination, retinoscopy, and refraction
- Referral for appropriate nephrology and hearing evaluation

Treatment

- Refractive correction
- Amblyopia management
- Pharmacologic pupillary dilation for small opacities
- Cataract extraction if visually significant opacity
- Clear lensectomy if unable to improve vision with refractive correction or pupillary dilation
- Treatment of underlying systemic nephrology disease
- Hearing loss management

Prognosis

- Good vision is possible with early diagnosis, close observation, and cataract extraction when indicated.

REFERENCES

Flinter F. Alport's syndrome. *J Med Genet.* 1997;34:326–330.

Savige J, Sheth S, Leys A, et al. Ocular features in Alport syndrome: pathogenesis and clinical significance. *Clin J Am Soc Nephrol.* 2015;10(4):703–709.

Trivedi R, Wilson ME. Anterior lenticonus in Alport syndrome. In: Wilson ME, Trivedi R, Pandey S, eds. *Pediatric Cataract Surgery; Techniques, Complications, and Management.* Philadelphia, PA: Lippincott Williams & Wilkins; 2005:194–198.

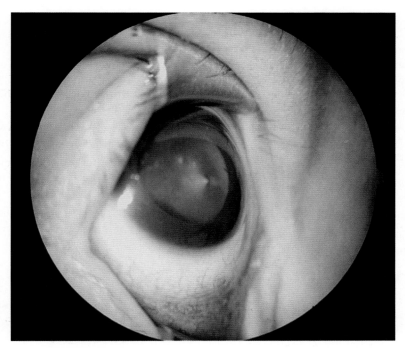

FIGURE 5-3. **Anterior lenticonus.**

POSTERIOR LENTICONUS

Posterior lenticonus is a thinning of the posterior capsule with an associated posterior bowing of the central lens capsule and cortical material (Fig. 5-4). Posterior lens opacification is progressive and can become full posterior subcapsular cataracts. Often at the time of cataract surgery, there is an associated hole in the posterior capsule that may lead to vitreous prolapse during surgery.

Etiology

- Congenital
- Hereditary (X-linked or autosomal dominant)

Symptoms

- Often no early symptoms
- Decreased vision with progression

Signs

- Oil-droplet sign on red reflex test
- Posterior lens changes seen on slit-lamp examination
- Amblyopia
- Irregular or high lenticular astigmatism
- Partial or complete opacification of visual axis
- Variable degrees of leukocoria

Diagnosis

- Detailed history, including family history
- Complete eye examination, including visual acuity, slit-lamp examination, dilated fundoscopic examination, retinoscopy, and refraction

Treatment

- Observation if small (less than 2–3 mm)
- Amblyopia management
- Refractive correction
- Cataract extraction if visually significant, with or without intraocular lens
- Clear lensectomy if unable to improve vision with refractive correction or dilation
- Special care to manage posterior capsule during surgery as most patients likely have capsular defect
- Given that this can be progressive, continued monitoring is recommended even if visually insignificant at diagnosis

Prognosis

- Congenital posterior lenticonus has a guarded but potentially good prognosis.
- Acquired or progressive posterior lenticonus can have a good prognosis.

REFERENCES

Amaya L, Taylor D, Russell-Eggitt I, et al. The morphology and natural history of childhood cataracts. *Surv Ophthalmol.* 2003;48:125–144.

Khali M, Saheb N. Posterior lenticonus. *Ophthalmology.* 1984;91:1429–1430.

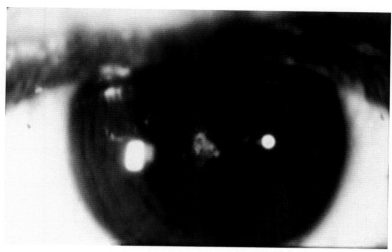

FIGURE 5-4. Posterior lenticonus: posterior lens opacification. Initially, this may not be visually significant, but it may progress to complete posterior subcapsular opacity.

SPHEROPHAKIA

Spherophakia occurs when the lens has a spherical shape instead of the normal biconvex shape. This causes increased lens thickness, increased curvature, and forward lens displacement with resultant lenticular myopia. Microspherophakia is when the lens is spherical and small. This is associated with the increased risk of dislocation (ectopia lentis) (Fig. 5-5).

Etiology

- Idiopathic or congenital
- Weill-Marchesani syndrome
- Marfan syndrome

Symptoms

- Mild to severely decreased visual acuity caused by progressive or acute changes in refractive error.
- Pain associated with pupillary block glaucoma

Signs

- High lenticular myopia
- Irregular astigmatism
- Amblyopia
- Pupillary block glaucoma
- Anterior or posterior lens dislocation

Diagnosis

- Detailed history to determine the etiology with special attention to systemic and family history
- Full ocular examination, including visual acuity, slit-lamp examination, and dilated fundoscopic examination
- Appropriate genetic or metabolic testing

Treatment

- Refractive correction
- Amblyopia management
- Lensectomy with postoperative aphakic glasses or contact lenses
- Lensectomy with intraocular lens if possible
- Treatment of secondary ocular conditions (i.e., pupillary block glaucoma)
- Refer to appropriate specialist for evaluation and treatment of underlying medical condition.

REFERENCES

Jensen AD, Cross HE, Paton D. Ocular complications in the Weill-Marchesani syndrome. *Am J Ophthalmol.* 1974;77:261–269.

Pikkel J, Irena E. Isolated spherophakia and glaucoma. *Case Rep Med.* 2013;2013:516490.

Ritch R, Chang BM, Liebmann JM. Angle closure in younger patients. *Ophthalmology.* 2003;110:1880–1889.

ACKNOWLEDGMENT

Jonathan H. Salvin and Hillary Gordon are acknowledged for their work and contributions in the writing of this chapter.

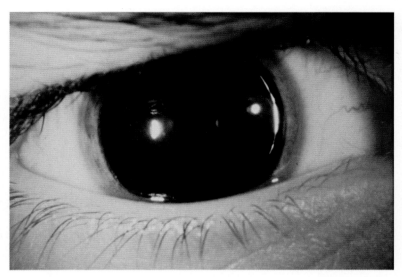

FIGURE 5-5. Microspherophakia. Patient with microspherophakia. The small and spherical lens edge is visible nasally. (Courtesy of Alex Levin, MD.)

Pediatric Uveitis

Kara C. LaMattina and Debra A. Goldstein ■

INTRODUCTION

Pediatric uveitis is a rare entity, accounting for anywhere from 5% to 10% of uveitis cases in tertiary referral centers. Although it is uncommon, it is an important condition as it presents diagnostic and therapeutic challenges and carries significant risk of morbidity. Children are often asymptomatic in diseases like juvenile idiopathic arthritis (JIA)–associated uveitis and may be preverbal and unable to express symptoms, both of which can lead to a delay in diagnosis. Diagnosis may also be delayed because children can be more difficult to examine than adults. In addition to the morbidities seen in adults (cataract, band keratopathy, glaucoma, cystoid macular edema [CME]), children also carry the risk of amblyopia, which may limit topical treatment options. They may also have unique side effects of systemic steroids, including growth retardation, which can further limit therapeutic options.

JUVENILE IDIOPATHIC ARTHRITIS

The most common systemic disease associated with pediatric uveitis, JIA is arthritis of unknown etiology with onset before age 16 with persistence for more than 6 weeks. The classification criteria as proposed by the International League of Associations for Rheumatology (ILAR) are outlined below.

Epidemiology and Etiology

Oligoarthritis

- Accounts for 50% to 60% of cases of JIA

- Involves four or fewer joints within the first 6 months of disease onset (usually knees, ankles, and fingers)

- Peak age of onset is 2 to 4 years

- Uveitis affects 30% to 50% of patients

- More common in females

- Subtypes include persistent (involves four or fewer joints throughout the disease course) and extended (may involve more than four joints after the first 6 months)

Polyarticular Rheumatoid Factor–Positive

- More than four joints involved in the first 6 months
- Accounts for ~2% of cases of JIA
- Mean age of onset between 9 and 12 years
- Rarely develop uveitis

Polyarticular Rheumatoid Factor–Negative

- More than four joints involved in the first 6 months
- Accounts for 20% to 30% of cases of JIA
- Bimodal age of onset: 1 to 3 years and 9 to 14 years
- Uveitis affects 5% to 10% of patients

Psoriatic Arthritis

- Arthritis with psoriasis, or arthritis with two or more of the following: dactylitis, nail pitting or onycholysis, psoriasis in a first-degree relative
- Accounts for ~5% of cases of JIA
- Bimodal age of onset: 1 to 2 years and 8 to 12 years
- Uveitis affects 10% to 20% of patients

Enthesitis-Related Arthritis

- Arthritis and enthesitis, or arthritis or enthesitis with two or more of the following: sacroiliac joint tenderness or inflammatory lumbosacral pain, HLA-B27 positivity, arthritis in a male after 6 years of age, ankylosing spondylitis, enthesitis-related arthritis, sacroiliitis with inflammatory bowel disease (IBD), reactive arthritis, or acute anterior uveitis in a first-degree relative
- Mean age of onset >10 years
- Affects boys more frequently than girls
- Uveitis affects 10% to 15% of patients

Systemic Arthritis

- Accounts for 10% of cases of JIA
- Mean age of onset <5 years
- No gender predilection
- Associated with fever, rash, lymphadenopathy, hepatosplenomegaly, pericarditis, peritonitis
- Can affect hip, cervical spine, temporomandibular joints
- Uveitis affects <1% of patients

Undifferentiated Arthritis

- Includes arthritis that does not fulfill inclusion criteria for a category, or fulfills criteria for more than one category
- Accounts for 5% to 10% of cases of JIA

Symptoms

- Uveitis associated with oligoarthritis is typically asymptomatic (screening is required).
- Polyarticular rheumatoid factor–negative JIA also tends to be asymptomatic (screening is required).
- Uveitis associated with enthesitis-related arthritis typically presents with pain, redness, and photophobia and usually affects one eye at a time, as in adult HLA-B27–positive patients (screening is not required).

Signs

Oligoarthritis

- Typically bilateral, nongranulomatous anterior uveitis
- Anterior chamber cell/flare ± anterior vitreous cell
- May develop band keratopathy, posterior synechiae, anterior synechiae, pupillary membranes (Fig. 6-1)
- Can be complicated by cataract, glaucoma, macular edema, hypotony

Enthesitis-Related Arthritis

- Severe acute anterior uveitis (often with fibrin and hypopyon, Fig. 6-2)
- Children with IBD may present with acute or chronic anterior uveitis, scleritis, CME, or retinal vasculitis

Differential Diagnosis

- Early-onset sarcoidosis/Blau syndrome
- Tubulointerestitial nephritis and uveitis (TINU)
- Post infectious uveitis

Diagnostic Evaluation

- Antinuclear antibody (ANA) in children with asymptomatic anterior uveitis
- HLA-B27 in patients with acute symptomatic anterior uveitis
- Workup for TINU, especially with bilateral acute anterior uveitis (urine β_2 microglobulin as screening test, see below)
- Workup for sarcoidosis (chest x-ray)
- Regular screening for uveitis of patients with JIA (see **Tables 6-1** and **6-2**)

Treatment

- Limit topical and systemic corticosteroids.
- Early initiation of systemic immunomodulatory therapy is associated with better visual outcomes (methotrexate is the most frequent first-line agent).

Prognosis

- Depends on the extent of disease on presentation.
- Generally good if diagnosed early and appropriate aggressive therapy is instituted.
- Outcomes are better with early initiation of steroid-sparing immunomodulatory therapy.

TABLE 6-1. American Academy of Pediatrics Guidelines for the Ophthalmological Screening of Children with JIA

JIA Subtype	Age of Onset	
	<7 y	>7 y
Pauciarticular		
ANA(+)	Every 3–4 mo	Every 6 mo
ANA(−)	Every 6 mo	Every 6 mo
Polyarticular		
ANA(+)	Every 3–4 mo	Every 6 mo
ANA(−)	Every 6 mo	Every 6 mo
Systemic	Every 12 mo	Every 12 mo

ANA, antinuclear antibody; JIA, juvenile idiopathic arthritis. Reprinted with permission from American Academy of Pediatrics Section on Rheumatology and Section on Ophthalmology. Guidelines for ophthalmologic examinations in children with juvenile rheumatoid arthritis. *Pediatrics.* 1993;92(2):295–296.

REFERENCES

Ernst BB, Lowder CY, Meisler DM, et al. Posterior segment manifestations of inflammatory bowel disease. *Ophthalmology.* 1991;98:1272–1280.

Gregory AC II, Kempen JH, Daniel E, et al; Systemic Immunosuppressive Therapy for Eye Diseases Cohort Study Research Group. Risk factors for loss of visual acuity among patients with uveitis associated with juvenile idiopathic arthritis: the Systemic Immunosuppressive Therapy for Eye Diseases Study. *Ophthalmology.* 2013;120(1):186–192.

Hafner R, Michels H. Psoriatic arthritis in children. *Curr Opin Rheumatol.* 1996;8:467–472.

Heiligenhaus A, Niewerth M, Ganser G, et al; German Uveitis in Childhood Study Group. Prevalence and complications of uveitis in juvenile idiopathic arthritis in a population-based nation-wide study in Germany: suggested modification of the current screening guidelines. *Rheumatology.*2007;46:1015–1019.

Kesen MR, Setlur V, Goldstein DA. Juvenile idiopathic arthritis-related uveitis. *Int Ophthalmol Clin.* 2008;48:21–38.

Kotaniemi K, Kaipiainen-Seppänen O, Savolainen A, et al. A population-based study on uveitis in juvenile rheumatoid arthritis. *Clin Exp Rheumatol.* 1999;17:119–122.

Levy-Clarke GA, Nussenblatt RB, Smith JA. Management of chronic pediatric uveitis. *Curr Opin Ophthalmol.* 2005;16:281–288.

Petty RE, Smith JR, Rosenbaum JT. Arthritis and uveitis in children: a pediatric rheumatology perspective. *Am J Ophthalmol.* 2003;135:879–884.

Petty RE, Southwood TR, Manners P, et al; International League of Associations for Rheumatology. International League of Associations for Rheumatology classification of juvenile idiopathic arthritis, second revision, Edmonton, 2001. *J Rheumatol.* 2004;31:390–392.

Stoll ML, Zurakowski D, Nigrovic LE, et al. Patients with juvenile psoriatic arthritis comprise two distinct populations. *Arthritis Rheum.* 2006;54(11):3564–3572.

Wu EY, Van Mater HA, Rabinovich CE. Juvenile idiopathic arthritis. In: Kliegman R, Stanton B, Schor N, St. Geme J, Behrman R, eds. *Nelson Textbook of Pediatrics.* 19th ed. Philadelphia, PA: Elsevier Health Sciences; 2011:829–838.

Zierhut M, Michels H, Stübiger N, et al. Uveitis in children. *Int Ophthalmol Clin.* 2005;45(2):135–156.

TABLE 6-2. Recommendations for Screening Based on the ILAR Classification of JIA

JIA Subtype	ANA	Age at Onset of JIA (y)	Duration of JIA (y)	Screening (mo)
Oligoarthritis	+	≤6	≤4	3
RF-negative polyarthritis				
Psoriatic arthritis	+	≤6	>4	6
Undifferentiated arthritis	+	≤6	≥7	12
	+	>6	≤2	6
	+	>6	>2	12
	−	≤6	≤4	6
	−	≤6	>4	12
	−	>6	NA	12
Enthesitis-related arthritis	NA	NA	12	
RF-positive polyarthritis	NA	NA	12	
Systemic arthritis	NA	NA	12	

ANA, antinuclear antibody; ILAR, International League of Associations for Rheumatology; JIA, juvenile idiopathic arthritis; RF, Rheumatoid Factor.

Reprinted with permission from Heiligenhaus A, Niewerth M, Ganser G, Heinz C, Minden K; German Uveitis in Childhood Study Group. Prevalence and complications of uveitis in juvenile idiopathic arthritis in a population-based nation-wide study in Germany: suggested modification of the current screening guidelines. *Rheumatology.* 2007;46:1015–1019.

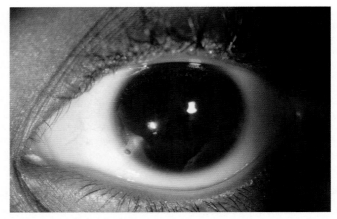

FIGURE 6-1. Juvenile idiopathic arthritis. Band keratopathy and posterior synechiae in a 7-year-old girl with juvenile idiopathic arthritis.

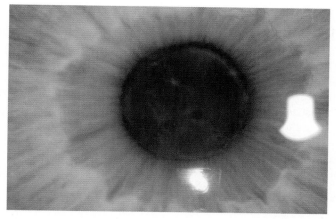

FIGURE 6-2. Enthesitis-associated uveitis. Fibrin membrane in a patient with enthesitis-associated acute anterior uveitis.

TUBULOINTERSTITIAL NEPHRITIS AND UVEITIS

Accounting for 15% to 20% of acute kidney injury, acute tubulointerstitial nephritis is frequently drug induced (about 70% of cases). This disease entity was first linked to uveitis in 1975 and accounts for 1% to 2% of all uveitis in tertiary referral centers. Uveitis may develop between 2 months before to 14 months after the onset of systemic symptoms (median 3 months after).

Epidemiology and Etiology

- Mean age of onset 15 years
- Conflicting reports on gender predilection
- Accounts for 1.1% to 2% of all pediatric uveitis in published literature, but true prevalence may be higher.

Symptoms

- Systemic: fever, weight loss, fatigue, malaise, anorexia, weakness, arthralgias, myalgias
- May have abdominal or flank pain
- Ocular: pain, redness, blurred vision, photophobia

Signs

- Predominantly bilateral, anterior, nongranulomatous inflammation
- Posterior findings (including vitritis, pars plana exudates, retinal vascular sheathing, intraretinal hemorrhages and exudates, focal chorioretinitis, and multifocal choroiditis) are seen in at least 20% of patients (Figs. 6-3 and 6-4).

Differential Diagnosis

- Early-onset sarcoidosis/Blau syndrome
- Post infectious uveitis
- JIA-associated uveitis

Diagnostic Evaluation

- Urine β_2 microglobulin
- Renal function (blood urea nitrogen, creatinine)

- HLA-DRB1
- May require kidney biopsy for definitive diagnosis

Treatment

- Topical and systemic corticosteroids
- May require immunomodulatory therapy if unable to wean off steroids

Prognosis

- Generally favorable with appropriate therapy
- Kidney disease usually self-limited, eye disease typically more chronic

REFERENCES

Dobrin RS, Vernier RL, Fish FJ. Acute eosinophilic interstitial nephritis and renal failure with bone marrow-lymph node granulomas and anterior uveitis. *Am J Med.* 1975;596:325–333.

Howarth L, Gilvert RD, Bass P, et al. Tubulointerstitial nephritis and uveitis in monozygotic twin boys. *Pediatr Nephrol.* 2004;19:917–919.

Kump LI, Cervantes-Castaneda RA, Androudi SN, et al. Analysis of pediatric uveitis cases at a tertiary referral center. *Ophthalmology.* 2005;112:1287–1292.

Levinson RD, Park MS, Rikkers SM, et al. Strong associations between specific HLA-DQ and HLA-DR alleles and the tubulointerstitial nephritis and uveitis syndrome. *Invest Ophthalmol Vis Sci.* 2003;44:653–657.

Mackensen F, Billing H. Tubulointerstitial nephritis and uveitis syndrome. *Curr Opin Ophthalmol.* 2009;20(6):525–531.

Mandeville JT, Levinson RD, Holland GN. The tubulointerstitial nephritis and uveitis syndrome. *Surv Ophthalmol.* 2001;46:195–208.

Raghavan R, Eknoyan G. Acute interstitial nephritis—a reappraisal and update. *Clin Nephrol.* 2014;82(3):149–162.

Rosenbaum JT. Bilateral anterior uveitis and interstitial nephritis. *Am J Ophthalmol.* 1988;105:534–537.

Smith JA, Mackensen F, Sen HN, et al. Epidemiology and course of disease in childhood uveitis. *Ophthalmology.* 2009;116(8):1544–1551.

Vohra S, Eddy A, Levin AV, et al. Tubulointerstitial nephritis and uveitis in children and adolescents. Four new cases and a review of the literature. *Pediatr Nephrol.* 1999;13:426–432.

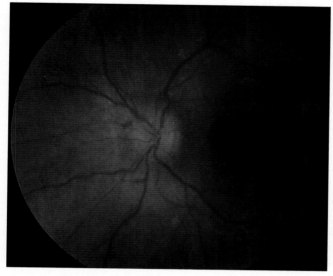

FIGURE 6-3. Tubulointerstitial nephritis and uveitis. Neovascularization of the disc in a 10-year-old boy with tubulointerstitial nephritis and uveitis.

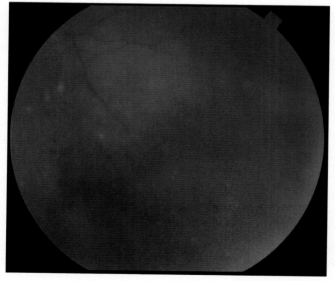

FIGURE 6-4. Tubulointerstitial nephritis and uveitis. Peripheral granulomas and vitreous hemorrhage in a 10-year-old boy with tubulointerstitial nephritis and uveitis.

BLAU SYNDROME/ EARLY-ONSET SARCOIDOSIS

Blau syndrome (also known as Blau-Jabs syndrome) is the autosomal-dominant familial form of early-onset sarcoidosis, with both entities characterized by granulomatous dermatitis, polyarthritis, and uveitis, with absence of the lung disease typically seen in sarcoidosis. Both diseases are correlated with *NOD2* mutations, although early-onset sarcoidosis is associated with a sporadic mutation. Both typically first present in children younger than age 4. There are two other subsets of pediatric sarcoidosis—infantile-onset panniculitis with uveitis and systemic granulomatosis and pediatric-onset "adult-type" sarcoidosis—which are not associated with this mutation. The pediatric-onset adult-type sarcoidosis tends to occur in early adolescence, with lung involvement in 90% to 100%.

Epidemiology and Etiology

- Systemic onset between the ages of 2 and 4 years
- Uveitis affects 60% to 80% of patients
- Uveitis occurs at a mean age of 4 years
- Accounts for 1.1% to 4.7% of cases of pediatric uveitis

Symptoms

- Skin (typically first manifestation): fine, scaly, erythematous, maculopapular rash on trunk/extremities
- Polyarthritis of metacarpal-phalangeal, metatarsal-phalangeal, and proximal-interphalangeal joints of hands and feet
- May also have wrist, knee, ankle, and elbow involvement
- Pain, redness, blurred vision, photophobia

Signs

- Bilateral, chronic, or recurrent granulomatous anterior or posterior uveitis
- Mutton-fat keratic precipitates (KP)
- May have anterior uveitis, intermediate uveitis, chorioretinitis, periphlebitis, macular edema, vein occlusion, optic neuropathy (Figs. 6-5 and 6-6)

Differential Diagnosis

- JIA-associated uveitis
- Pediatric-onset adult-type sarcoidosis
- Tuberculosis

Diagnostic Evaluation

- Skin biopsy shows noncaseating epithelioid and giant-cell granulomas
- Testing for CARD15/NOD2 mutations

Treatment

- Limited topical and systemic steroids
- Systemic immunomodulatory therapy with antimetabolites and/or biologic agents (often needed)

Prognosis

- Generally good, although posterior complications can lead to moderate to severe vision loss

REFERENCES

Blau EB. Familial granulomatous arthritis, iritis, and rash. *J Pediatr.* 1985;107:689–693.

Hoffmann AL, Milman N, Byg KE. Childhood sarcoidosis in Denmark 1979–1994: incidence, clinical features and laboratory results at presentation in 48 children. *Acta Paediatr.* 2004;93:30–36.

Jabs DA, Houk JL, Bias QB, et al. Familial granulomatous synovitis, uveitis, and cranial neuropathies. *Am J Med.* 1985;78(5):801–804.

Kanazaaw N, Matsushima S, Kambe N, et al. Presence of a sporadic case of systemic granulomatosis syndrome with a CARD15 mutation. *J Invest Dermatol.* 2004;122(3):851–852.

Khairallah M, Attia S, Zaouali S, et al. Pattern of childhood-onset uveitis in a referral center in Tunisia, North Africa. *Ocul Immunol Inflamm.* 2006;14(4):225–231.

Kump LI, Cervantes-Castaneda RA, Androudi SN, et al. Analysis of pediatric uveitis cases at a tertiary referral center. *Ophthalmology.* 2005;112:1287–1292.

Miceli-Richard C, Lesage S, Rybojad M, et al. Card15 mutations in Blau syndrome. *Nat Genet.* 2001;29(1):19–20.

Petty RE, Laxer RM, Lindsley CB, et al. *Textbook of Pediatric Rheumatology.* Philadelphia, PA: Elsevier Saunders; 2016:517–525.

Rahimi M, Oustad M, Ashrafi A. Demographic and clinical features of pediatric uveitis at a tertiary referral center in Iran. *Middle East Afr J Ophthalmol.* 2016;23(3):237–240.

Raiji VR, Miller MM, Jung LK. Uveitis in Blau syndrome from a de novo mutation of the NOD2/CARD15 gene. *J AAPOS.* 2011;15:205–207.

Rose CD, Doyle TM, McIlvain-Simpson G, et al. Blau syndrome mutation of CARD15/NOD2 in sporadic early onset granulomatous arthritis. *J Rheumatol.* 2005;32(2):373–375.

Rosé CD, Pans S, Casteels I, et al. Blau syndrome: cross-sectional data from a multicenter study of clinical, radiological and functional outcomes. *Rheumatology (Oxford).* 2015;54(6):1008–1016.

Smith JA, Mackensen F, Sen HN, et al. Epidemiology and course of disease in childhood uveitis. *Ophthalmology.* 2009;116(8):1544–1551.

Vaphiades MS, Eggenberger E. Childhood sarcoidosis. *J Neuroophthalmol.* 1998;18(2):99–101.

Wouters CH, Maes A, Foley KP, et al. Blau syndrome, the prototypic auto-inflammatory granulomatous disease. *Pediatr Rheum Online J.* 2014;12:33.

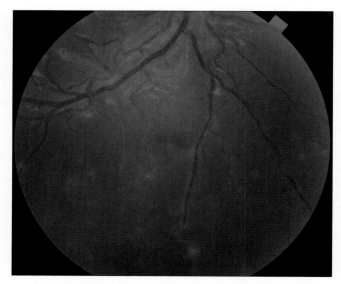

FIGURE 6-5. **Blau syndrome.** Periphlebitis in a 17-year-old girl with Blau syndrome.

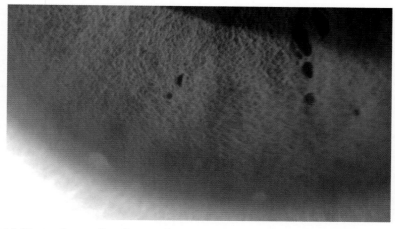

FIGURE 6-6. **Blau syndrome.** Granulomatous keratic precipitates in a child with Blau syndrome.

POST INFECTIOUS AUTOIMMUNE UVEITIS

Most commonly seen after group A streptococcal infection, post infectious autoimmune uveitis typically occurs 1 to 6 weeks after systemic illness with bilateral anterior uveitis.

Epidemiology and Etiology

- Mean age 10.9 years
- Accounts for ~7% of cases of pediatric uveitis

Symptoms

- Flu-like illness and sore throat
- Blurred vision, pain, photophobia

Signs

- Acute bilateral anterior uveitis
- +/− CME, papillitis

Differential Diagnosis

- JIA-associated uveitis
- Tubulointerstitial nephritis and uveitis
- Early-onset sarcoidosis/Blau syndrome

Diagnostic Evaluation

- Serum antistreptolysin O titers (if continuing to rise may require further antibiotic therapy)

Treatment

- Appropriate antibiotic therapy
- Topical steroid therapy is usually adequate.

Prognosis

- Excellent, usually self-limited

REFERENCES

Benjamin A, Tufail A, Holland GN. Uveitis as the only clinical manifestation of post streptococcal syndrome. *Am J Ophthalmol.* 1997;123(2)258–260.

Birnbaum AD, Jiang Y, Vasaiwala R, et al. Bilateral simultaneous-onset nongranulomatous acute anterior uveitis: clinical presentation and etiology. *Arch Ophthalmol.* 2012;130(11):1389–1394.

Gallagher MJ, Muqit MM, Jones D, et al. Post-streptococcal uveitis. *Acta Ophthalmol Scand.* 2006;84(3):424–428.

Holland GN. Recurrent anterior uveitis associated with streptococcal pharyngitis in a patient with a history of post-streptococcal syndrome. *Am J Ophthalmol.* 1999;27:345–347.

Paroli MP, Spinucci G, Liverani M, et al. Uveitis in childhood: an Italian clinical and epidemiological study. *Ocul Immunol Inflamm.* 2009;17(4):238–242.

Ur Rehman S, Anand S, Reddy A, et al. Poststreptococcal syndrome uveitis: a descriptive case series and literature review. *Ophthalmology.* 2006;113(4)701–706.

TRAUMATIC UVEITIS

Mild unilateral ocular inflammation is often seen after blunt trauma.

Epidemiology and Etiology

- Males are more commonly affected (70%–79%).
- Mean age 31 ± 16.5 years
- Typically unilateral disease

Symptoms

- Pain, redness, photophobia

Signs

- Miosis
- Ciliary flush
- Decreased intraocular pressure
- +/− Hyphema

Differential Diagnosis

- JIA-associated uveitis: enthesitis subtype (HLA-B27-associated anterior uveitis)
- Sarcoidosis

Diagnostic Evaluation

- Gonioscopy
- Ultrasound if suspicion of foreign body
- If inflammation is severe or persistent, consider etiologies other than trauma.

Treatment

- Topical corticosteroids
- Topical cycloplegics

Prognosis

- Excellent if no concomitant traumatic nerve/retinal damage, usually self-limited

REFERENCES

Engelhard SB, Patrie J, Prenshaw J, et al. Traumatic uveitis in the mid-Atlantic United States. *Clin Ophthalmol.* 2015;9:1869–1874.

Rosenbaum JT, Tammaro J, Robertson JE Jr. Uveitis precipitated by nonpenetrating ocular trauma. *Am J Ophthalmol.* 1991;112(4)392–395.

HERPESVIRIDAE

Accounting for up to 30% of infectious uveitis, herpes viruses (including varicella zoster, herpes simplex, and cytomegalovirus) can cause uveitis affecting both the anterior and posterior segments.

Epidemiology and Etiology

- No gender predilection
- Accounts for 1.5% to 6.2% of cases of pediatric uveitis
- May have history of perinatal exposure or chickenpox

Symptoms

- Redness, pain, photophobia, blurred vision

Signs

- Dendritiform corneal lesion
- Interstitial keratitis (Fig. 6-7)
- Mild-moderate anterior chamber reaction
- White or pigmented, granulomatous or stellate KP (often diffuse and not confined to Arlt triangle)
- Sectoral or patchy iris atrophy
- Elevated intraocular pressure
- Retinal necrosis and vasculitis, in cases with posterior involvement

Differential Diagnosis

- Fuchs heterochromic iridocyclitis
- JIA-associated uveitis: enthesitis subtype
- Toxoplasmosis

Diagnostic Evaluation

- All patients need a dilated fundus examination to rule out retinitis.
- Consider anterior chamber tap with polymerase chain reaction (PCR) in cases where diagnosis is unclear.

Treatment

- Systemic antivirals
- Topical corticosteroids

Prognosis

- Generally very good for anterior uveitis, depends on severity of retinitis in cases with posterior involvement

REFERENCES

Barron BA, Gee L, Hauck WW, et al. Herpetic Eye Disease Study. A controlled trial of oral acyclovir for herpes simplex stromal keratitis. *Ophthalmology.* 1994;101(12):1871–1872.

Hettinga YM, de Groot-Mijnes JD, Rothova A, et al. Infectious involvement in a tertiary center pediatric uveitis cohort. *Br J Ophthalmol.* 2015;99(1):103–107.

Khairallah M, Attia S, Zaouali S, et al. Pattern of childhood-onset uveitis in a referral center in Tunisia, North Africa. *Ocul Immunol Inflamm.* 2006;14(4):225–231.

Kump LI, Cervantes-Castaneda RA, Androudi SN, Foster CS. Analysis of pediatric uveitis cases at a tertiary referral center. *Ophthalmology.* 2005;112:1287–1292.

Rahimi M, Oustad M, Ashrafi A. Demographic and clinical features of pediatric uveitis at a tertiary referral center in Iran. *Middle East Afr J Ophthalmol.* 2016;23(3):237–240.

Siverio Júnior CD, Imai Y, Cunningham ET Jr. Diagnosis and management of herpetic anterior uveitis. *Int Ophthalmol Clin.* 2002;42(1):43–48.

Van der Lelij A, Ooijman FM, Kijlstra A, Rothova A. Anterior uveitis with sectoral iris atrophy in the absence of keratitis: a distinct clinical entity among herpetic eye diseases. *Ophthalmology.* 2000;107(6):1164–1170.

Wilhelmus KR, Gee L, Hauck WW, et al. Herpetic Eye Disease Study. A controlled trial of topical corticosteroids for herpes simplex stromal keratitis. *Ophthalmology.* 1994;101(12):1883–1895.

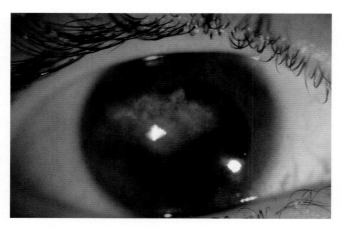

FIGURE 6-7. **Herpes keratitis.** Herpetic interstitial keratitis in a young girl.

PARS PLANITIS

Pars planitis is a form of intermediate uveitis with no known infectious or inflammatory etiology. There is a risk of developing multiple sclerosis (MS).

Epidemiology and Etiology

- Mean age of onset 8 to 10 years
- Male predominance (57%–84%)
- Accounts for 17% to 20.8% of cases of pediatric uveitis

Symptoms

- Floaters, blurred vision
- Photophobia in cases with concurrent anterior uveitis

Signs

- Usually bilateral (asymmetric) involvement
- May present with strabismus or amblyopia
- Mild-moderate anterior chamber reaction
- Vitreous cell
- Snowbanks and snowballs (Figs. 6.8 and 6.9)
- Periphlebitis

Differential Diagnosis

- MS-associated intermediate uveitis
- Sarcoidosis
- Syphilis
- Tuberculosis

Diagnostic Evaluation

- Neurologic review of systems with magnetic resonance imaging as indicated to rule out MS
- Consider ultrasound if fundus exam is limited by vitritis

Treatment

- Topical, periocular, and systemic steroids
- May require systemic immunomodulatory therapy
- Tumor necrosis factor inhibitors: consider risk of MS
- Pars plana vitrectomy with laser (or cryo) peripheral retinal ablation

Prognosis

- Dependent on development of complications (cataract, glaucoma, CME, vitreous hemorrhage, retinoschisis, retinal detachment)
- Good if caught early in the disease course and appropriately treated

REFERENCES

Giuliari GP, Chang PY, Thakuria P, Hinkle DM, Foster CS. Pars plana vitrectomy in the management of paediatric uveitis: the Massachusetts Eye Research and Surgery Institution experience. *Eye (Lond)*. 2010;24(1):7–13.

Jain R, Ferrante P, Reddy GT, et al. Clinical features and visual outcome of intermediate uveitis in children. *Clin Exp Ophthalmol*. 2005;33:22–25.

Kump LI, Cervantes-Castañeda RA, Androudi SN, Foster CS. Analysis of pediatric uveitis cases at a tertiary referral center. *Ophthalmology*. 2005;112:1287–1292.

Malalis JF, Bhat P, Shapiro M, et al. Retinoschisis in pars planitis. *Ocul Immunol Inflamm*. 2017;25:344–348.

Maris K, Van Castler J, Wouters C, et al. Clinical symptoms and complications of pars planitis in childhood. *Bull Soc Belge Ophthalmol*. 2005;295:29–33.

Nikkhah H, Ramezani A, Ahmadieh H, et al. Childhood pars planitis: clinical features and outcomes. *J Ophthalmic Vis Res*. 2011;6(4):249–254.

Paroli MP, Spinucci G, Liverani M, Monte R, Pezzi PP. Uveitis in childhood: an Italian clinical and epidemiological study. *Ocul Immunol Inflamm*. 2009;17(4):238–242.

Romero R, Peralta J, Sendagorta E, Abelairas J. Pars planitis in children: epidemiologic, clinical, and therapeutic characteristics. *J Pediatr Ophthalmol Strabismus*. 2007;44:288–293.

Smith JA, Mackensen F, Sen HN, et al. Epidemiology and course of disease in childhood uveitis. *Ophthalmology*. 2009;116(8):1544–1551.

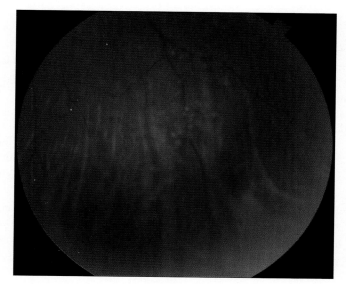

FIGURE 6-8. **Pars planitis.** Snowballs in an 8-year-old boy with pars planitis.

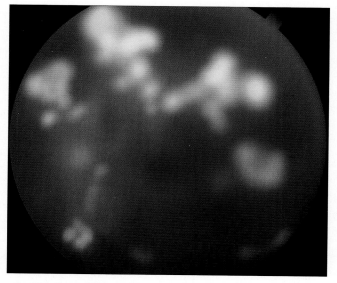

FIGURE 6-9. **Pars planitis.** Very active pars planitis in a 10-year-old girl.

TOXOPLASMOSIS

*T*oxoplasma gondii is an intracellular parasite that can be transmitted congenitally or acquired postnatally. Postnatal infection is generally caused by consumption of contaminated water, undercooked meat, or exposure to cat feces, as cats serve as the definitive host of the parasite.

Epidemiology and Etiology

- Most common cause of posterior uveitis in children
- Accounts for 3.3% to 25.6% of all pediatric uveitis
- Affects up to 1 in 770 live-born infants in endemic regions
- Mean age 9.5 ± 4.4 years
- No gender predilection
- Bilateral in 30% to 63.5% of cases, although disease tends to be active in one eye at a time

Symptoms
- Blurred/poor vision, redness, floaters

Signs
- Microcephaly, hydrocephalus, microphthalmia (congenital infection)
- Strabismus
- Acute anterior and intermediate uveitis (not typical in neonates)
- Retinitis with or without adjacent chorioretinal scars (Figs. 6-10 to 6-12)
- Papillitis
- Retinal vasculitis
- Intraocular pressure (IOP) often elevated at presentation

Differential Diagnosis
- Behçet disease
- Acute retinal necrosis
- Pars planitis
- Endophthalmitis

Diagnostic Evaluation
- Diagnosis is typically made clinically.
- PCR of vitreous or aqueous fluid in atypical cases

Treatment
- Antiparasitics (e.g., trimethoprim/sulfamethoxazole, azithromycin, pyrimethamine) with or without topical and/or systemic corticosteroids
- Congenital infection is treated in collaboration with pediatrician for the first year of life with sulfadiazine, pyrimethamine, and folinic acid.

Prognosis
- Dependent on location

REFERENCES

Garza-Leon M, Garcia LA. Ocular toxoplasmosis: clinical characteristics in pediatric patients. *Ocul Immunol Inflamm.* 2012;20(2):130–138.

Hettinga YM, de Groot-Mijnes JD, Rothova A, de Boer JH. Infectious involvement in a tertiary center pediatric uveitis cohort. *Br J Ophthalmol.* 2015;99(1):103–107.

Kump LI, Cervantes-Castaneda RA, Androudi SN, Foster CS. Analysis of pediatric uveitis cases at a tertiary referral center. *Ophthalmology.* 2005;112:1287–1292.

Pivetti-Pezzi P. Uveitis in children. *Eur J Ophthalmol.* 1996;6:293–298.

Rahimi M, Oustad M, Ashrafi A. Demographic and clinical features of pediatric uveitis at a tertiary referral center in Iran. *Middle East Afr J Ophthalmol.* 2016;23(3):237–240.

Smith JA, Mackensen F, Sen HN, et al. Epidemiology and course of disease in childhood uveitis. *Ophthalmology.* 2009;116(8):1544–1551.

Standford MR, Tan HK, Gilbert RE. Toxoplasmic retinochoroiditis presenting in childhood: clinical findings in a UK survey. *Br J Opthhalmol.* 2006;90:1464–1467.

Vasconcelos-Santos DV, Machado Azevedo DO, Campos WR, et al. Congenital toxoplasmosis in Southeastern Brazil: results of early ophthalmologic examination of a large cohort of neonates. *Ophthalmology.* 2009;116(11):2199–2205.

Wallon M, Kodjikian L, Binquet C, et al. Long-term ocular prognosis in 327 children with congenital toxoplasmosis. *Pediatrics.* 2004;113(6):1567–1572.

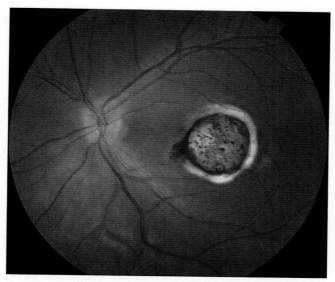

FIGURE 6-10. Congenital toxoplasmosis. Macular scar in a 12-year-old girl with congenital toxoplasmosis.

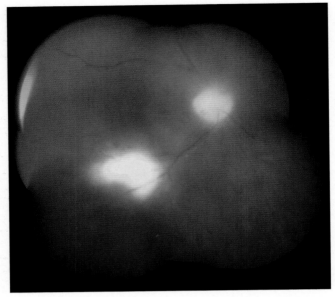

FIGURE 6-11. Active acquired toxoplasmosis. Note the white patch of retinitis, vitreous haze, and vasculitis.

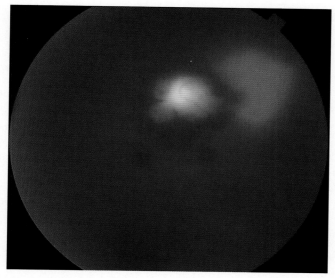

FIGURE 6-12. **Recurrent toxoplasmosis.** Recurrent toxoplasmosis with active white retinitis adjacent to old scar.

TOXOCARIASIS

Toxocariasis is most commonly caused by *Toxocara canis*, a roundworm carried by dogs and shed in the feces, and *Toxocara cati*, a roundworm carried by cats. It is typically acquired by ingestion of contaminated food or water.

Epidemiology and Etiology

- Mean age of onset 6 years
- Accounts for 0.3% to 7.4% of cases of pediatric uveitis

Symptoms

- Blurred vision, pain, photophobia
- Flashes, floaters
- Asymptomatic

Signs

- Leukocoria
- Retinal granuloma in peripheral retina or posterior pole (Fig. 6-13)
- Endophthalmitis
- Vitritis, vitreous strands
- Tractional retinal detachment
- Typically unilateral

Differential Diagnosis

- Tuberculosis
- Sarcoidosis
- Toxoplasmosis
- Retinoblastoma

- Pars planitis

Diagnostic Evaluation

- Serum titers

Treatment

- Topical and systemic corticosteroids
- Can treat systemic disease with antiparasitics, but generally not indicated for isolated ocular involvement (parasite assumed to be dead when patient presents with eye disease)

Prognosis

- Depends on localization, but generally unilateral, so does not result in bilateral visual impairment

REFERENCES

Hettinga YM, de Groot-Mijnes JD, Rothova A, de Boer JH. Infectious involvement in a tertiary center pediatric uveitis cohort. *Br J Ophthalmol.* 2015;99(1):103–107.

Khairallah M, Attia S, Zaouali S, et al. Pattern of childhood-onset uveitis in a referral center in Tunisia, North Africa. *Ocul Immunol Inflamm.* 2006;14(4):225–231.

Kump LI, Cervantes-Castaneda RA, Androudi SN, Foster CS. Analysis of pediatric uveitis cases at a tertiary referral center. *Ophthalmology.* 2005;112:1287–1292.

Liu Y, Zhang Q, Li J, Ji X, Xu Y, Zhao P. Clinical characteristics of pediatric patients with ocular toxocariasis in China. *Ophthalmologica.* 2016;235(2):97–105.

Paroli MP, Spinucci G, Liverani M, Monte R, Pezzi PP. Uveitis in childhood: an Italian clinical and epidemiological study. *Ocul Immunol Inflamm.* 2009;17(4):238–242.

Rahimi M, Oustad M, Ashrafi A. Demographic and clinical features of pediatric uveitis at a tertiary referral center in Iran. *Middle East Afr J Ophthalmol.* 2016;23(3):237–240.

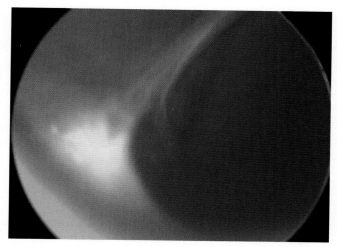

FIGURE 6-13. Toxocariasis. Peripheral retinal toxocara lesion in a 10-year-old boy with falciform retinal fold.

TUBERCULOSIS

Caused by the airborne pathogen *Mycobacterium tuberculosis*, tuberculosis can affect multiple organ systems.

Epidemiology and Etiology

- Accounts for 0.3% to 0.5% of cases of pediatric uveitis

Symptoms

- Pain, redness, photophobia
- Blurred vision
- Flashes, floaters

Signs

- Granulomatous anterior inflammation: mutton-fat KP, iris nodules
- Broad-based posterior synechiae
- Vitritis
- Single or multiple choroidal tubercles
- Serpiginous-like choroiditis
- Periphlebitis

Differential Diagnosis

- Sarcoidosis
- Syphilis
- Vogt-Koyanagi-Harada disease

Diagnostic Evaluation

- Tuberculin skin test, such as purified protein derivative
- Interferon gamma release assay such as QuantiFERON gold
- Chest x-ray (limit computed tomography scan use to reduce radiation exposure in pediatric population)

Treatment

- Four-drug therapy (rifampin, isoniazid, ethambutol, and pyrazinamide) for 2 months followed by 4 to 9 months of therapy with rifampin and isoniazid, typically managed by infectious disease specialist
- Topical and systemic corticosteroids
- May require addition of systemic immunomodulatory therapy

Prognosis

- Depends on localization (posterior segment disease may be aggressive and poorly responsive to therapy)

REFERENCES

Cutrufello NJ, Karakousis PC, Fishler J, Albini TA. Intraocular tuberculosis. *Ocul Immunol Inflamm.* 2010;18(4):281–291.

Gupta A, Bansal R, Gupta V, Sharma A, Bambery P. Ocular signs predictive of ocular tuberculosis. *Am J Ophthalmol.* 2010;149(4):562–570.

Hettinga YM, de Groot-Mijnes JD, Rothova A, de Boer JH. Infectious involvement in a tertiary center pediatric uveitis cohort. *Br J Ophthalmol.* 2015;99(1):103–107.

Paroli MP, Spinucci G, Liverani M, Monte R, Pezzi PP. Uveitis in childhood: an Italian clinical and epidemiological study. *Ocul Immunol Inflamm.* 2009;17(4):238–242.

Patel SS, Saraiya NV, Tessler HH, Goldstein DA. Mycobacterial ocular inflammation: delay in diagnosis and other factors impacting morbidity. *JAMA Ophthalmol.* 2013 Jun;131(6):752–758.

IDIOPATHIC UVEITIS

Idiopathic uveitis is a diagnosis of exclusion and can present as anterior, intermediate, posterior, or panuveitis. It accounts for anywhere from 21.5% to 50% of pediatric uveitis. Differential diagnosis depends on localization and clinical presentation, and treatment is based on location and severity of uveitis.

REFERENCES

Friling R, Kramer M, Snir M, Axer-Siegel R, Weinberger D, Mukamel M. Clinical course and outcome of uveitis in children. *J AAPOS.* 2005;9(4):379–382.

Khairallah M, Attia S, Zaouali S, et al. Pattern of childhood-onset uveitis in a referral center in Tunisia, North Africa. *Ocul Immunol Inflamm.* 2006;14(4):225–231.

Smith JA, Mackensen F, Sen HN, et al. Epidemiology and course of disease in childhood uveitis. *Ophthalmology.* 2009;116(8):1544–1551.

Tugal-Tutkun I, Havrlikova K, Power WJ, Foster CS. Changing patterns in uveitis of childhood. *Ophthalmology.* 1996;103(3):375–383.

MASQUERADES

I t is important to note that neoplasms such as leukemia and retinoblastoma can present with pseudohypopyon, spontaneous hyphema, or iris masses that may be misdiagnosed as uveitis. The pseudohypopyon is typically creamy (leukemia) or chalky (retinoblastoma) white in color. The iris masses are larger and may be less well-defined than inflammatory iris nodules and may be vascularized. Another disorder that could be mistaken for uveitis is juvenile xanthogranuloma (JXG), which typically presents with unilateral, flesh-colored iris nodules. Diagnosis in all cases requires high clinical suspicion; leukemia can be diagnosed with anterior-chamber paracentesis and cytologic examination. Diagnosis of JXG may require tissue biopsy.

REFERENCES

Croxatto JO, Fernandez MR, Malbran ES. Retinoblastoma masquerading as ocular inflammation. *Ophthalmologica.* 1983;186(1):48–53.

Fontanilla FA, Edward DP, Wong M, Tessler HH, Eagle RC, Goldstein DA. Juvenile xanthogranuloma masquerading as melanoma. *J AAPOS.* 2009;13(5):515–518.

Rowan PJ, Sloan JB. Iris and anterior chamber involvement in leukemia. *Ann Ophthalmol.* 1976;8(9):1081–1085.

Schwartz LW, Rodrigues MM, Hallett JW. Juvenile xanthogranuloma diagnosed by paracentesis. *Am J Ophthalmol.* 1974;77(2):243–246.

Tahan SR, Pastel-Levy C, Bhan AK, Mihm MC Jr. Juvenile xanthogranuloma. Clinical and pathologic characterization. *Arch Pathol Lab Med.* 1989;113(9):1057–1061.

Wolintz AH, Goldstein JH, Seligman BR, Rosner F, Wesely AC, Lee SL. Secondary glaucoma in leukemia. *Ann Ophthalmol.* 1969;82(6):771–773.

Zakka KA, Yee RD, Shorr N, Smith GS, Pettit TH, Foos RY. Leukemic iris infiltration. *Am J Ophthalmol.* 1980;89(2):204–209.

Congenital Abnormalities of the Optic Nerve

Aldo Vagge and Leonard B. Nelson ◼

OPTIC NERVE HYPOPLASIA

- Optic nerve hypoplasia (ONH) is a congenital, nonprogressive developmental abnormality in which the optic nerve is smaller than usual because of reduced numbers of retinal ganglion cells. It is frequently associated with other central nervous system (CNS) abnormalities.

- ONH may be unilateral or bilateral (80%) and may be asymmetric.

- Most common congenital optic disc anomaly

- Optic nerve aplasia is rare. No pupillary light reflex and absence of the optic disc, nerve fiber layer, and retinal blood vessels on examination.

Etiology

- Not completely understood

- Parental drug and alcohol abuse contributes to an increasing prevalence of ONH. Drug associations include exposure to carbemazepine, isotretinoin, phenytoin, quinine, and valproic acid. Young maternal age and maternal insulin-dependent diabetes have also been implicated in some cases (associated with subtype—superior segmental optic hypoplasia).

Genetics

- Most cases are sporadic.

- Bilateral ONH is inherited in an autosomal-dominant pattern based on the few families reported. Mutation in the *PAX6* (11q13) gene is responsible.

- Mutation in the *HESX1* gene has been identified in sporadic septo-opto dysplasia and pituitary disease.

- Mutation in the *TUBA8* gene is associated with polymicrogyria and ONH.

Symptoms

- Decreased vision in one or both eyes

- Strabismus may be associated with unilateral ONH.

Signs

- Range of visual acuity is 20/20 to no light perception since vision is determined primarily by the integrity of the papillomacular nerve fibers more than the overall size of the disc.

● Amblyopia as a result of accompanying strabismus and anisometropia

● Nystagmus: often develops at 1 to 3 months of age in bilateral cases

● Strabismus may be associated with unilateral ONH.

● Afferent pupil defect in asymmetric or unilateral cases

● Visual fields (VFs) often have localized defects as well as general constriction.

● Abnormally small optic nerve head, often gray or pale in color with "double-ring sign" (scleral canal surrounds a small optic nerve) (Fig. 7-1)

● Superior segmental hypoplasia of the optic nerve is a segmental form of ONH occurring in some children of insulin-dependent diabetic mother.

● Retinal vascular tortuosity is common.

Associated Conditions

● Septa-optic dysplasia: combination of small anterior visual pathways, absence of the septum pellucid, and thinning or agenesis of the corpus callosum

● Endocrine dysfunction: pituitary gland abnormalities in approximately 15% of patients with ONH. Patients are at risk for hypothalamic and pituitary dysfunction such as growth hormone deficiency (most common), hypothyroidism, hyperprolactinemia, panhypopituitarism, and diabetes insipidus.

● Cerebral anomalies such as error in hemispheric migration (schizencephaly, cortical heterotopias) or hemispheric injury (periventricular leukomalacia [PVL], encephalomalacia). PVL can be associated with another form of ONH characterized by large optic cups and a thin neuroretinal rim contained within normal-sized optic discs. This occurs secondary to trans-synaptic degeneration of optic axons caused by bilateral lesions in the optic radiations.

● Developmental delay more common in patients with bilateral ONH, highly correlated with corpus callosum hypoplasia and hypothyroidism

Diagnostic Evaluation

● Magnetic resonance imaging (MRI) to rule out CNS malformations

● Refer to a pediatric endocrinologist if patients show clinical signs of endocrine dysfunction or pituitary abnormalities on MRI. Pediatrician should follow growth chart for endocrine changes. Undiagnosed endocrine deficiencies are at risk for impaired growth, hypoglycemia, seizures, and death.

● Automated VF testing may be useful but children are often too young to cooperate.

Differential Diagnosis

● Optic atrophy

● Optic nerve coloboma

● Ocular albinism

Treatment

● No treatment available to improve the vision in ONH

● Correction of refractive errors

● Treatment for superimposed amblyopia

● Surgery for concurrent strabismus or nystagmus may be considered.

● Consider polycarbonate eye glasses for protection of the better-seeing eye.

Prognosis

● Visual acuity is generally nonprogressive. Complications are in general related to endocrinopathies and CNS malformations.

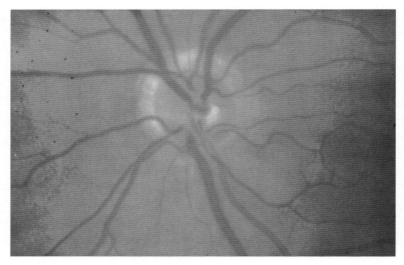

FIGURE 7-1. **Optic nerve hypoplasia.** Note the double-ring sign.

MORNING GLORY DISC ANOMALY

- Morning glory disc anomaly (MGDA) is a rare, congenital, usually unilateral funnel-like excavation of the posterior fundus that incorporates the optic disc.
- The name derives from the similarity to the morning glory flower.
- More common in female and rare in African Americans.

Etiology

- The embryologic basic of MGDA is unclear. A defect in fetal fissure closure or a primary mesenchymal abnormality has been hypothesized as embryonic origins of morning glory anomaly.

Symptoms

- Decreased vision most common in the involved eye
- Color vision defect

Signs

- Visual acuity can range from normal vision to no light perception but in general is approximately 20/100 to 20/200.
- Strabismus
- Leucokoria
- Amblyopia
- Myopia
- Afferent pupil defect
- VF defects, commonly enlarged blind spots
- The optic disc is markedly enlarged, orange or pink in color, with a surrounding annular ring of pigmented uveal tissues. Retinal vessels increased in number emanate radially

from the disc, a central white tuft of glial tissue. Macula may be incorporated into the excavation (macular capture) (Fig. 7-2).

- Serous retinal detachment (RD) in one-third of patients

Associated Conditions

- Trans-sphenoidal basal encephalocele associated with midfacial anomalies (hypertelorism, flat nasal bridge, midline notch in the upper lip, and sometimes a midline cleft in the soft palate).
- Midline or other brain abnormalities (e.g., agenesis of the corpus callosum, pituitary abnormalities)
- Ipsilateral abnormalities of the carotid circulation such as stenosis or aplasia of the carotid arteries with or without Moyamoya syndrome (progressive stenosis of the terminal portion of the internal carotid artery and its main branches)
- Associated with ipsilateral orofacial hemangioma—this association may fall within the spectrum of the PHACE syndrome (posterior fossa malformation, large facial hemangioma, arterial anomalies, cardiac anomalies and aortic coarctation, and eye anomalies)
- Associated with neurofibromatosis type 2
- MGDA has been described as part of the spectrum of renal coloboma syndrome.

Diagnostic Evaluation

- MRI and magnetic resonance angiography should be obtained to rule out brain and vascular abnormalities.
- Rule out endocrine dysfunction (thyroid-stimulating hormone and growth hormone levels) and kidney involvement (basic metabolic panel and urinalysis)

Differential Diagnosis

- Optic nerve coloboma
- Peripapillary staphyloma

Treatment

- No treatment available to improve the vision in MGDA
- Correction of refractive errors

- Treatment for amblyopia if associated
- RD is usually addressed with pars plana vitrectomy and long-standing gas tamponade.

Prognosis

- Vision is usually stable unless RD occurs. Optic neuritis and progressive optic atrophy have been documented.

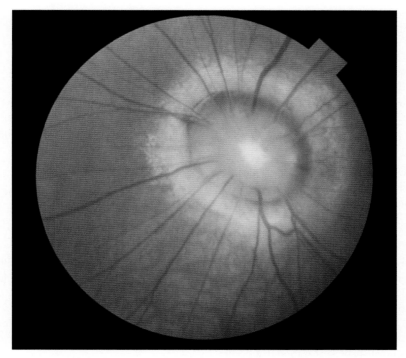

FIGURE 7-2. **Morning glory disc.** Morning glory disc anomaly showing an enlarged excavation, abnormal retinal vascular pattern, annular pigmentation surrounding the nerve head, and central glial tuft and peripapillary changes. (Courtesy of Alex Levin, MD.)

OPTIC DISC COLOBOMA

- Clearly demarcated bowl-shaped excavation of the optic disc, which is typically decentered and deeper inferiorly.
- Unilateral and bilateral optic disc coloboma occur with similar frequencies.
- Occasionally involvement of the entire disc occurs.
- Other types of uveal coloboma can coexist.
- They may be isolated or part of a systemic syndrome.

Etiology

- Thought to result from incomplete or abnormal fusion of the two sides of the proximal end of the embryonic fissure
- Most cases are sporadic but may be autosomal dominant, autosomal recessive, or X-linked recessive.
- A wide variety of mutations have been documented in patients with coloboma—*CHD7* mutation is associated with 60% of cases of CHARGE syndrome.

Symptoms

- Visual acuity may be mildly or severely decreased in one or both eyes—the degree of foveal involvement by the coloboma is the only feature that relates to visual outcome.

Signs

- White, bowl-shaped excavation that occurs in an enlarged optic disc. The excavation is decentered inferiorly and the superior neuroretinal rim is relatively spared. In case of complete excavation of the entire disc, the excavation is deeper inferiorly.
- Chorioretinal coloboma can be associated—if so, microphthalmia is frequently present
- Iris and ciliary body colobomas often coexist.
- Rhegmatogenous or serous RD may develop in some patients—rhegmatogenous

are often associated when chorioretinal coloboma, whereas serous detachment is more common in case of isolated optic nerve coloboma.

Associated Conditions

- CHARGE association: coloboma, choanal atresia, congenital heart disease, and multiple other abnormalities
- Walker-Warburg syndrome
- Goltz focal dermal hypoplasia
- Aicardi syndrome
- Goldenhar sequence
- Linear sebaceous nevus syndrome
- Dandy-Walker malformation
- Renal coloboma syndrome—with a mutation of PAX2 transcription
- Microphthalmia—in case of chorioretinal involvement

Diagnostic Evaluation

- Optical coherence tomography (OCT) has been useful in observing the intercalary membrane that covers the chorioretinal defect and is continuous with the neural retina.
- A complete systemic evaluation is important to rule out other associated anomalies.

Differential Diagnosis

- MGDA
- Peripapillary staphyloma

Treatment

- No specific treatment is available for optic disc coloboma
- Treatment for amblyopia, if associated
- Optimal refractive correction may be indicated.
- RD surgery as indicated

Prognosis

- Vision is usually stable unless RD occurs

OPTIC DISC PITS

- Optic disc pit (ODP) is an oval or round excavation of variable color, depth, and location in the optic disc.
- The temporal optic disc side is the most commonly involved.
- Often unilateral, although bilateral cases have been reported in 15% of the cases.
- They are rare, with an estimated incidence of 1 in 11,000 people.

Etiology

- It is not entirely clear—they are thought to result from an imperfect closure of the superior edge of the embryonic fissure.
- Histologically, an ODP is a herniation of dysplastic retina into a collagen-rich excavation that extends into the subarachnoid space through a defect in the lamina cribrosa.
- The pathogenesis of the macular changes is still controversial—the fluid may be vitreous fluid, cerebrospinal fluid, leakage from blood vessels at the base of the pit, or leakage from the choroid. Also, serous macular detachment is caused by direct communication between the optic pit and the subretinal space or from the optic pit and retina. In the latter case, fluid may move into the retina, causing a schisis-like separation of the inner and outer layers, with the neurosensory serous RD occurring secondary to this schisis. In addition, vitreous traction appears to be an important factor in the pathogenesis of optic pit–related macular detachment.
- ODPs are generally sporadic, although familial occurrence has been reported as a dominant trait.

Symptoms

- Optic pits are asymptomatic unless there is subretinal fluid—approximately 45% of the eyes develop serous macular detachment usually in the second or third decades of life. When subretinal fluid is present, visual acuity decreases to 20/40–20/60.

Signs

- ODPs are usually seen as single, oval-shaped depressions at the optic disc. They are most commonly found at the inferotemporal aspect of the optic disc, but may also be found elsewhere, including centrally. Usually they are gray, white, or yellowish in color (**Fig. 7-3**).
- The signs associated with ODP maculopathy include intraretinal and subretinal fluid accumulation, and retinal pigment changes.
- Amblyopia in children especially in eye with serous macular detachment

Associated Conditions

- Rarely associated with basal encephalocele

Diagnostic Evaluation

- OCT to evaluate the subretinal fluid—typically OCT may show a schisis-like separation between the inner and outer retina.
- VF—arcuate scotoma is most common
- Intravenous fluorescein angiography (IVFA) is helpful in the differential diagnosis of serous detachment.
- Amsler grid can be used to monitor the macular involvement.

Differential Diagnosis

- Optic disc anomalies such as choroidal and scleral crescent
- Tilted disc syndrome (TDS)
- Circumpapillary staphyloma
- Hypoplastic disc
- Glaucomatous optic neuropathy
- Central serous retinopathy and subretinal neovascular membranes for serous macular detachment

Treatment

- No treatment is required for an isolated optic pit.

- Laser photocoagulation (between the area of the serous RD and the optic disc), macular buckling, and a combination of posterior vitrectomy, photocoagulation, and gas tamponade are the commonly used procedures for the treatment of ODP maculopathy. Less-invasive treatments like laser photocoagulation should be tried initially.

Prognosis

- Isolated ODP has usually an excellent prognosis.

- Associated retinal complications such as serous macular detachment can be progressive and decrease significantly visual acuity—advice patients about the importance of regular comprehensive eye exams and the use of Amsler grid testing.

- Posterior macular reattachment can occur in rare instances.

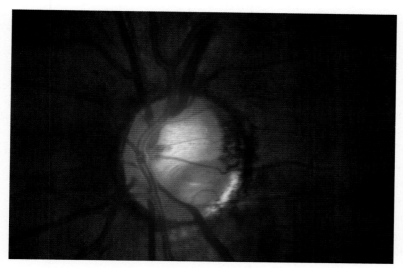

FIGURE 7-3. Optic disc pit. Congenital pit of the optic nerve head.

TILTED DISC SYNDROME

- TDS is a congenital, nonhereditary bilateral condition where the optic nerve appears to enter the eye in an oblique angle.

- Elevated superior pole of the optic disc with posterior displacement of the inferior nasal disc resulting in an oval appearance of the optic nerve head

- Often accompanied by:
  - Scleral crescent located inferiorly and inferonasally (**Fig. 7-4**)
  - Situs inversus of retinal vessel
  - Posterior ectasia of the inferonasal retina and choroid

- Typically associated with myopic astigmatism because of the fundus abnormalities (posterior ectasia)

Etiology

- Unknown, but may have some pathogenic relationship with colobomatous defect.

Symptoms

- Best corrected visual acuity (BCVA) may be reduced.

Signs

- Myopic astigmatism

- Tilted disc with associated features as previously described

- VF defects are often associated with complete bitemporal hemianopia that does not respect the midline. Repeat perimetry after addition of a −4.00 lens often eliminates the VF abnormalities (refractive nature of the defects). In some cases, VF defects persist despite refractive correction due to an abnormal inferonasal ectasia. However, TDS has been reported with true bilateral hemianopsia and congenital suprasellar brain tumor.

- Amblyopia

Associated Conditions

- Suprasellar brain tumors

- Tilted disc without retinal ectasia occurs in patients with trans-sphenoidal encephalocele.

- Craniofacial anomalies such as hypertelorism, Crouzon syndrome, and Alport syndrome have been observed in association with tilted disc.

- Other conditions reported with tilted disc are:
  - Ehler-Danlos type III
  - Hemifacial atrophy
  - Congenital horizontal gaze palsy
  - Familial dextrocardia
  - Exotropia

Diagnostic Evaluation

- Refraction and dilated fundus exam—diagnosis can be made based on the fundoscopic appearance of the optic disc.

- VF often shows complete bitemporal hemianopia that does not respect the midline (unlike chasmal lesions).

- MRI brain in any patient with TDS and VF defects to rule out suprasellar tumors

Differential Diagnosis

- ONH
- Optic nerve coloboma
- Peripapillary staphyloma
- Papilledema

Treatment

- No medical treatment for the primary disorder

- Appropriate refractive error correction

- Amblyopia therapy as indicated may improve nonorganic visual loss.

Prognosis

- Broad range of BCVA

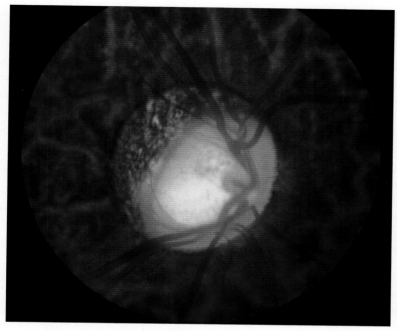

FIGURE 7-4. Tilted disc. Note the temporal scleral crescent.

PERIPAPILLARY STAPHYLOMA

- Peripapillary staphyloma is a generally sporadic, rare, usually unilateral optic disc anomaly characterized by a deep excavation of the area of the fundus surrounding the optic disc.
- Optic disc head sits at the base of the posterior pole excavation.
- Not associated with glial or vascular abnormalities of the disc, uveal coloboma, and progression
- Affected eyes typically are emmetropic or slightly myopic, although high myopia has been reported.

Etiology

- The etiology is unknown. It appears to arise as incomplete differentiation of sclera. Staphyloma may be the consequence of the development of normal intraocular pressure causing scleral herniation.

Symptoms

- Visual acuity is usually mildly or severely reduced.

Signs

- Peripapillary staphyloma is usually associated with a relatively normal appearance of the optic disc.
- Centrocecal scotomas commonly occur in eyes with decreased vision.

Associated Conditions

- Usually absence of associated systemic abnormalities or intracranial diseases

- Peripapillary staphyloma has been reported to be associated with basal encephalocele in patients with midfacial abnormalities.
- PHACE syndrome, linear nevus sebaceous syndrome, and 18q-syndrome have been observed in association with peripapillary staphyloma.
- Nystagmus, strabismus, and head turn
- Increased risk of RD

Diagnostic Evaluation

- Ocular ultrasound and electroretinogram (ERG) can help the diagnosis especially in pediatric patients.
- OCT can be used to evaluate a peripapillary staphyloma.
- VF can show a centrocecal scotoma especially in eyes with decreased vision.
- MRI of the brain is indicated for children with midfacial abnormalities.

Differential Diagnosis

- MGDA
- Optic disc coloboma
- TDS

Treatment

- No medical treatment for the primary disorder
- Amblyopia therapy and strabismus surgery as needed
- RD surgery as indicated
- Consider polycarbonate eye glasses.

Prognosis

- Risk of RD

OPTIC DISC DRUSEN (PSEUDOPAPILLEDEMA)

- Optic disc drusen are acellular calcific deposits located within the optic nerve head.
- Optic drusen are typically buried in the optic disc early in life and become more superficial later.
- Often bilaterally
- Most common form of pseudopapilledema—anomalous elevation of the optic disc unrelated to increased intracranial pressure

Etiology

- The etiology is unknown—they are thought to result by a disturbance in axonal metabolism with slowed axoplasmic flow, congenitally dysplastic discs with a propensity for drusen formation, or a small scleral canal that physically compresses the optic nerve, causing ganglion cell death, with extrusion and calcification of mitochondria.
- Optic drusen may be transmitted as an irregular dominant trait—they are frequently familial.

Symptoms

- Usually asymptomatic with no visual complaints
- Rarely (especially in children) transient visual obscuration—probably secondary to transient disc ischemia

Signs

- Disc is often elevated and its margins are blurred and obscured.
- Disc vessel is clearly visible, without hyperemia, dilated capillaries, or venous congestion.
- Absence of exudates and cotton wool spots

- Retinal vasculature of eyes is frequently anomalous—higher frequency of cilioretinal arteries
- Afferent pupillary defect and acquired dyschromatopsia may be present and they are signs of an optic neuropathy.
- VF can show peripheral defects that tend to increase in frequency with increasing age. The progression is generally slow. The most common VF defects are nasal defect, concentric constriction, and enlarged blind spot.
- Peripapillary or disc hemorrhage, choroidal neovascular membrane (CNVM), nonarteritic anterior ischemic optic neuropathy (NAION), and retinal artery or vein occlusion can be complications of optic disc drusen.

Associated Conditions

- Optic disc drusen have been reported in association with many ocular and systemic disorders.
- Space-occupying lesions have been harbored with optic disc drusen and progressive visual loss.
- The most commonly associated conditions are:
  - Retinitis pigmentosa
  - Pseudoxanthoma elasticum and angioid streaks
  - Alagille syndrome

Diagnostic Evaluation

- B scan ultrasonography: drusen appear with high reflectivity and posterior shadowing
- Fundus autofluorescence: drusen display autofluorescence (poor reliability in buried drusen)
- Fluorescein angiography: drusen stain in late stage. Helpful to distinguish between optic disc drusen and true optic disc edema

- OCT: focal hyper reflective mass posterior to the outer plexiform and outer nuclear layers, with loss of the inner and outer segment photoreceptor junction (poor reliability at distinguishing buried drusen vs. true optic disc edema)
- VF testing should be performed as soon as children can do so reliably.
- Orbital CT—calcification in optic disc
- MRI brain in any patient with associated progressive visual loss

Differential Diagnosis

- Optic neuritis
- Posterior scleritis
- Toxoplasmosis
- Idiopathic intracranial hypertension
- Ischemic optic neuropathy
- Compressive optic neuropathy
- Optic nerve infiltrates
- Papilledema
- Sarcoidosis
- Optic nerve tumors
- Leber hereditary optic neuropathy

Treatment

- Drusen alone need no medical therapy.

- CNVMs may require laser photocoagulation or intravitreal anti-VEGF.
- Ischemic complications (NAION and retinal vascular occlusions) managed in the absence of drusen

Prognosis

- Usually very good but complications can occur
- VF defects are identified in up to 51% of children and become more common with increasing age.
- Hemorrhagic complications—peripapillary or disc hemorrhage
- CNVM
- NAION
- Retinal artery or vein occlusion

REFERENCES

Dutton GN. Congenital disorders of the optic nerve: excavations and hypoplasia [review]. *Eye (Lond)*. 2004;18(11):1038–1048.

Hoyt C, Taylor D. *Pediatric Ophthalmology and Strabismus.* 4th ed. St. Louis, MO: Elsevier Saunders; 2013:543–560.

Maguire JI, Murchison AP, Jaeger EA. *Wills Eye Hospital 5-Minute Ophthalmology Consult.* Philadelphia, PA: Lippincott Williams & Wilkins; 2012.

Retinal Anomalies

BEST DISEASE

Barry N. Wasserman ■

Etiology

An autosomal dominant disorder also called vitelliform macular dystrophy, Best disease leads to retinal pigment epithelium (RPE) degeneration and secondary loss of photoreceptors in the macula. Mutations lead to abnormal bestrophin, a Ca^{2+} sensitive Cl^- channel protein. Lipofuscin accumulates in the RPE cells yielding a characteristic "egg yolk" appearance (hence the name vitelliform) in the fovea and macula. Multifocal lesions may also occur. Several genes have been identified, including the *BEST1* and *PRPH2*, which is associated with an adult form. In families negative for these genes, *IMPG1* and *IMPG2* genes have been identified as causal.

Symptoms

Early in the disease process, patients may be asymptomatic, but later metamorphopsia and decreased visual acuity occur. Symptoms are variable and may be asymmetric, with significant vision loss in adulthood.

Signs

Stages are described on the basis of phenotypic appearance in the macula, which may be asymmetric between the eyes. Early stage may only reveal subtle RPE mottling or may be normal. Later, yellow-orange material collects in the macula as a 0.5-to-5.0-mm-diameter lesion, yielding the classic "egg yolk" appearance. Clear fluid slowly builds around the lesion in the subretinal space, with resultant cystic appearance with fluid level (**Fig. 8-1A**). As this fluid dissipates, the lesion again changes to a more "scrambled egg" (vitelliruptive) stage, associated with pigment clumping (**Fig. 8-1B**). Later stages include atrophic changes with fibrosis, macular degeneration, and significant vision loss, followed sometimes with choroidal neovascularization.

Differential Diagnosis

- Stargardt disease
- Sorsby macular dystrophy
- Pattern dystrophy
- North Carolina macular dystrophy
- Solar retinopathy

- Coalescence of basal laminar drusen
- Central serous retinopathy with fibrinous exudate
- Pigment epithelial detachment of age-related macular degeneration
- Adult foveomacular dystrophy
- Age-related macular degeneration

Diagnostic Evaluation

Diagnosis is based on clinical findings, along with electrophysiologic studies revealing normal electroretinogram and abnormal electrooculogram. In addition, there is high autofluorescence. Optical coherence tomography (OCT) detects subretinal deposits and fluid. Genetic studies may reveal mutation in the bestrophin gene.

Treatment

No treatment for early disease, but late choroidal neovascularization has been treated with intravitreal injection of bevacizumab. Genetic counseling and examination of family members are recommended, as are low vision and occupational consultations.

Prognosis

Some patients maintain good vision (20/40) throughout life. In others, good vision (20/20 to 20/50) usually persists through the early stages but decreases to 20/200 in the fifth and sixth decades as the atrophic and cicatricial stages progress.

REFERENCES

Goodwin P. Hereditary retinal disease. *Curr Opin Ophthalmol.* 2008;19:255–262.

Leu J, Schrage NF, Degenring RF. Choroidal neovascularisation secondary to Best's disease in a 13-year-old boy treated by intravitreal bevacizumab. *Graefes Arch Clin Exp Ophthalmol.* 2007;245(11):1723–1725.

Meunier I, Manes G, Bocquet B, et al. Frequency and clinical pattern of vitelliform macular dystrophy caused by mutations of interphotoreceptor matrix *IMPG1* and *IMPG2* genes. *Ophthalmology.* 2014;121:2406–2414.

Spaide RF, Noble K, Morgan A, et al. Vitelliform macular dystrophy. *Ophthalmology.* 2006;113:1392–1400.

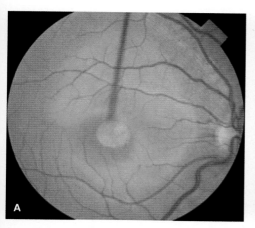 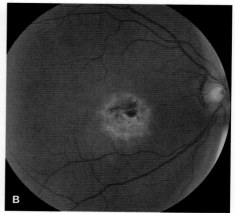

FIGURE 8-1. Best disease. A. Best disease with early macular "egg yolk" appearance. **B.** Best disease with later scrambled-egg appearance.

CHOROIDEREMIA

Barry N. Wasserman ■

Etiology

An X-linked recessive disease, choroideremia is a progressive retinal degeneration. Males carriers show loss of choriocapillaris and RPE. Female carriers can show mild signs of the disease, with patchy retinal abnormalities and corresponding visual field (VF) defects due to Lyonization, but are generally asymptomatic. Mutation in the *CHM* gene affects production of the Rab escort protein 1 (REP-1). Degeneration begins in the midperiphery and progresses centrally both toward the macula and toward the periphery.

Symptoms

Patients present in the first two decades of life with early loss of night vision and peripheral vision. Central vision may be maintained until around the fifth decade but is eventually lost.

Signs

Retinal examination reveals loss of the RPE and choriocapillaris, with exposure of the larger choroidal vessels (Fig. 8-2). Remaining RPE may have a salt-and-pepper appearance. Later in the disease, large areas of exposed sclera may be seen on fundoscopy. Posterior subcapsular cataracts may be associated.

Differential Diagnosis

● Advanced retinitis pigmentosa

● Gyrate atrophy

● Pathologic myopia

● Chorioretinitis (e.g., acute retinal necrosis, following cytomegalovirus [CMV] retinitis)

Diagnostic Evaluation

X-linked inheritance with typical fundus appearance is seen in male patients. VF testing demonstrates constriction. Fluorescein angiography reveals large choroidal vessels due to loss of overlying RPE and choriocapillaris. Electroretinogram may be consistent with a rod–cone dystrophy early in the disease but eventually becomes extinguished. Genetic analysis to assess mutation in the *CHM* gene may be performed, and analysis of peripheral blood is available to demonstrate absence of the Rab escort protein 1. Female carriers may demonstrate patches of irregular pigmentation in the RPE. SD-OCT may demonstrate reduced subfoveal choroidal thickness and increased foveal thickness as the disease progresses, despite unchanged visual acuity.

Treatment

Genetic counseling for family members should be suggested. Low vision evaluation and treatment may be helpful. Gene therapy has shown some success in animal models.

Prognosis

Patients progressively lose night and peripheral vision. Central vision is often maintained into adulthood but is ultimately lost.

REFERENCES

Kamron KN, Islam F, Moore AT, et al. Clinical and genetic features of choroideremia in childhood. *Ophthalmology.* 2016;123(10):2158–2165.

Lee TK, McTaggart KE, Sieving PA, et al. Clinical diagnoses that overlap with choroideremia. *Can J Ophthalmol.* 2003;38(5):364–372.

MacDonald IM, Russell L, Chan CC. Choroideremia: new findings from ocular pathology and review of recent literature. *Surv Ophthalmol.* 2009;54(3):401–407.

MacDonald IM, Smaoui N, Seabra MC. Choroideremia. In: Pagon RA, Bird TC, Dolan CR, Stephens K, eds. *GeneReviews* [Online]. Seattle: University of Washington; 2010.

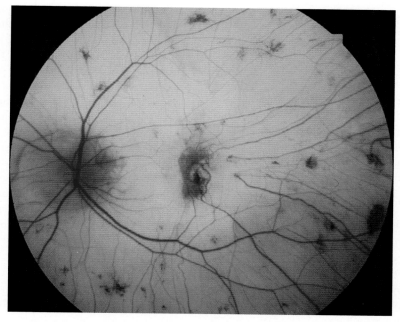

FIGURE 8-2. Choroideremia. Choroideremia at advanced stage, with complete loss of retinal pigment epithelium and choriocapillaris.

GYRATE ATROPHY

Barry N. Wasserman ■

Etiology

Gyrate atrophy is an autosomal recessive disease caused by the deficiency of the mitochondrial enzyme, ornithine aminotransferase. Elevated ornithine levels are toxic to the RPE, causing gradual loss of peripheral vision and night vision. Mutations of the ornithine aminotransferase gene (10q26) have been identified.

Symptoms

Nyctalopia and loss of visual field may begin in the first two decades but may not be manifest until the fifth decade. The disease affects both eyes symmetrically. Central vision is spared usually until the fourth or fifth decade but then declines. Symptoms and signs may vary widely in patients in all age groups.

Signs

Fundus examination early in the disease shows scalloped areas of geographic atrophic RPE and choriocapillaris (Fig. 8-3). The macula is relatively spared until late in the disease, though epiretinal membranes and cystoid macular edema can occur. Patients may have cataracts and myopia.

Differential Diagnosis

- Choroideremia
- Retinitis pigmentosa
- Choroidal atrophy
- Chorioretinitis (e.g., acute retinal necrosis, following CMV retinitis)

Diagnostic Evaluation

Ocular examination may reveal mildly decreased visual acuity, and refractive error is commonly myopic. Cataracts may be seen on slit-lamp evaluation. Fundoscopy shows midperipheral and peripheral scalloped geographic areas of RPE and choriocapillaris. Areas of intact RPE may have increased pigmentation. The macula is usually spared early in the disease, but cystoid macular edema may be demonstrated with OCT. Optic atrophy and attenuated retinal vessels are seen later in the disease. VFs are markedly constricted, and electroretinogram reveals absent photopic and scotopic responses. SD-OCT may demonstrate intraretinal cystic spaces and hyperreflective deposits in the ganglion cell layer. Outer retinal tubulations are round tubular, rosette-like structures found in the outer nuclear layer of some patients with advanced disease. Plasma ornithine levels are markedly elevated.

Treatment

Genetic counseling is suggested. A diet restricting arginine will lower the plasma ornithine and may slow the loss of visual function. Low vision services should be recommended.

Prognosis

Although dietary arginine restriction delays the loss of function, the macula is eventually affected in most patients.

REFERENCES

Kaiser-Kupfer MI, Caruso RC, Valle D, et al. Use of an arginine-restricted diet to slow progression of visual loss in patients with gyrate atrophy. *Arch Ophthalmol.* 2004;122:982–984.

Peltola KE, Nanto-Salonen K, Heinonen OJ, et al. Ophthalmologic heterogeneity in subjects with gyrate atrophy of choroid and retina harboring the L402P mutation of ornithine aminotransferase. *Ophthalmology.* 2001;108:721–729.

Sergouniotis PI, Davidson AE, Lenassi E, et al. Retinal structure, function, and molecular pathologic features in gyrate atrophy. *Ophthalmology.* 2012;119(3):596–605.

Tamara TL, Andrade RE, Muccioli C, et al. Cystoid macular edema in gyrate atrophy of the choroid and retina: a fluorescein angiography and optical coherence tomography evaluation. *Am J Ophthalmol.* 2005;140:147–149.

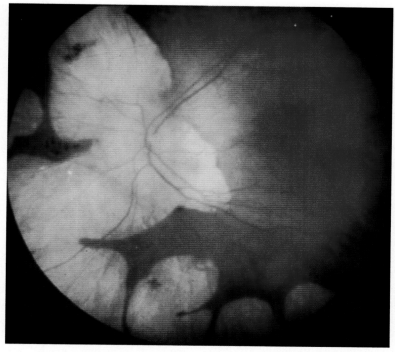

FIGURE 8-3. Gyrate atrophy. Gyrate atrophy with scalloped geographic atrophy of the retinal pigment epithelium and choriocapillaris. The macula is spared early in the disease.

LEBER CONGENITAL AMAUROSIS

Barry N. Wasserman ■

Etiology

Leber congenital amaurosis is a severe congenital retinal dystrophy affecting both cones and rods. Vision is often less than 20/200. Mutations in over 14 genes have been identified. The disease is mainly autosomal recessive and rarely autosomal dominant.

Symptoms and Signs

Patients present with nystagmus at 2 to 3 months of age. Children show poor visual behavior and some show self-stimulatory eye poking (oculodigital reflex). Pupils may be sluggish or paradoxical. Ophthalmoscopic findings are highly variable and may include a normal fundus appearance. Highly abnormal findings may also include chorioretinal atrophy, macular "coloboma" (**Fig. 8-4A**), retinal pigment epithelial irregularities, leopard spotting, nummular pigmentary abnormalities (**Fig. 8-4B**), and subretinal flecks. Retinal vessel attenuation and optic disc pallor are frequently present. Cataract, keratoconus, and strabismus may be associated findings.

Differential Diagnosis

- Achromatopsia
- Cone dystrophy
- Goldmann-Favre disease
- Refsum phytanic acid storage disease
- Bassen-Kornzweig (abetalipoproteinemia) syndrome
- Juvenile retinal dystrophy
- Toxoplasmosis (when macular "coloboma" is present)

Diagnostic Evaluation

Family history may reveal consanguinity or distantly related affected individuals. Examination including retinal evaluation, combined with extinguished electroretinogram findings, is diagnostic. Molecular genetic mutation screens are now available. Systemic and blood testing are important to rule out treatable causes, like Refsum phytanic acid storage disease. As there may be associated abnormalities of kidneys, liver, or hearing, appropriate testing is recommended.

Treatment

Low vision evaluation and treatment can aid in function in some patients. Gene transfer via subretinal administration of adeno-associated viral (AAV) vectors encoding has demonstrated safety and in some cases efficacy for patients with mutations in the gene *RPE65*. *RPE65* mutations account for 6% to 16% of Leber congenital amaurosis, and treatment with recombinant AAV vector expressing *RPE65* has not been associated with serious adverse events, and follow-up studies reveal durable improvement in some patients. The magnitude of improvement did decline with time in some patients in early studies.

Prognosis

Vision for most patients is poor. Future advances in gene therapy are promising.

REFERENCES

Goodwin P. Hereditary retinal disease. *Curr Opin Ophthalmol.* 2008;19:255–262.

Simonelli F, Maguire AM, Testa F, et al. Gene therapy for Leber's congenital amaurosis is safe and effective through 1.5 years after vector administration. *Mol Ther.* 2010;18(3):643–650.

Traboulsi EI. The Marshall M. Parks memorial lecture: making sense of early-onset childhood retinal dystrophies—the clinical phenotype of Leber congenital amaurosis. *Br J Ophthalmol.* 2010;94(10):1281–1287.

Weleber RG, Pennesi ME, Wilson DJ, et al. Results at 2 years after gene therapy for RPE65-deficient Leber congenital amaurosis and severe early childhood onset retinal dystrophy. *Ophthalmology.* 2016;123(7):1606–1620.

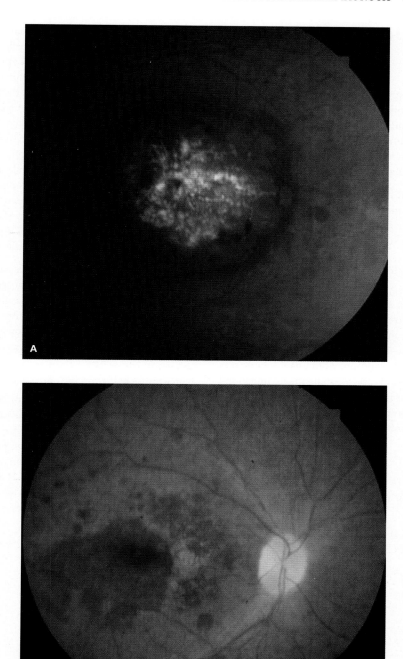

FIGURE 8-4. **Leber congenital amaurosis.** Leber congenital amaurosis with macular "coloboma" (**A**) and nummular pigmentary abnormalities (**B**).

ASTROCYTIC HAMARTOMA

Anuradha Ganesh ■

Retinal astrocytic hamartoma is a glial tumor arising from the retinal nerve fiber layer. It is most frequently associated with tuberous sclerosis (Bourneville disease) but may very rarely be seen in neurofibromatosis or as an isolated ocular finding in otherwise normal individuals.

Astrocytic hamartomas are believed to be congenital in most cases but may not be recognized until later in childhood. Patients with these lesions are usually asymptomatic.

Epidemiology and Etiology

Most astrocytic hamartomas occur congenitally in association with tuberous sclerosis, a phakomatosis characterized by the triad of seizures, mental retardation, and skin lesions. Tuberous sclerosis has an estimated incidence of 1 in 15,000 to 100,000 and exhibits autosomal dominant inheritance. About 60% of cases are spontaneous mutations. Mutations in either the *TSC1* or *TSC2* gene, on chromosomes 9q34 and 16p13, respectively, result in tuberous sclerosis (**Table 8-1**).

Signs

About 50% of patients with tuberous sclerosis develop astrocytic hamartomas, approximately

TABLE 8-1. Typical Manifestations of Tuberous Sclerosis

Skin lesions (<95% incidence)
Hypomelanotic macules
Facial angiofibromas (adenoma sebaceum)
Brain
Seizures (<90% incidence)
Developmental delay (<60% incidence)
Additional manifestations
Periungual fibromas
Pleural cysts and spontaneous pneumothorax
Renal angiomyolipoma
Cardiac rhabdomyoma
Hamartomas of the liver, thyroid, pancreas, or testis

50% of whom have bilateral involvement. Retinal astrocytic hamartomas are usually small, ranging from 0.5 to 5.0 mm in diameter, and are principally of two types. Small, flat, smooth tumors appear as subtle, ill-defined, semitranslucent thickening of the nerve fiber layer (**Fig. 8-5A**). Over time, they may become more opaque and contain calcification and may be associated with subretinal fluid and cystoid retinal edema. Larger, opaque, calcified, sessile, whitish-yellow nodular masses ("mulberry lesion") are found at the optic nerve (**Fig. 8-5B**). VF testing may reveal a scotoma in the area corresponding to the tumor. SD-OCT shows these lesions as "moth eaten" optically empty spaces arising from the nerve fiber layer.

Occasionally, lesions may produce vitreous hemorrhage, vitreous seeding, subretinal hemorrhage, or retinal detachment. Presence of yellow, lipoproteinaceous exudation in the sensory retina and subretinal space is an uncommon feature.

Less frequent ocular manifestations include patches of iris or RPE hypopigmentation and hamartomas of the iris and ciliary body.

Patients with an astrocytic hamartoma of the retina or optic nerve should be evaluated for tuberous sclerosis, which is characterized by the triad of skin lesions, seizures, and mental retardation. Additional manifestations include hamartomas in various organ systems. Diagnostic criteria for tuberous sclerosis facilitate identifying definite, probable, and possible cases.

Differential Diagnosis

- Retinoblastoma
- Retinocytoma
- Myelinated nerve fibers
- Retinal or optic nerve granuloma
- Drusen of the optic nerve
- Papillitis/papilledema
- Optic nerve infiltration (e.g., tuberculosis, sarcoid, leukemia)

Diagnostic Evaluation

- OCT: The astrocytic hamartoma replaces normal retinal architecture and appears as an optically hyperreflective mass with retinal disorganization, moth-eaten spaces, and posterior shadowing.

- Fluorescein angiography: The tumor appears relatively hypofluorescent in the arterial phase. Superficial find blood vessels are seen during the venous phase. The tumor stains intensely and homogeneously in the late phases. This test is rarely indicated.

- B-scan ultrasonography: A larger, calcified lesion often appears as a discrete, oval, solid mass with a sharp anterior border.

- Biopsy: In rare cases, differentiation from retinoblastoma (young patient) or choroidal melanoma (older patient) requires fine-needle aspiration biopsy.

- Imaging/ultrasonography: To detect astrocytomas in the brain and other parts of the body including chest and abdomen.

Treatment and Prognosis

Most cases of retinal astrocytoma are asymptomatic and do not require treatment. Rarely some tumors can exhibit aggressive behavior and cause hemorrhage, retinal detachment, and, even more uncommonly, neovascular glaucoma. Serial follow-up is indicated. Retinal detachment can be treated with demarcating laser photocoagulation. Progressive lesions may require measures such as endoresection, brachytherapy, and at times enucleation. Family members should be examined for manifestations of tuberous sclerosis. Genetic testing may be useful in confirming the diagnosis and identifying affected relatives, allowing for early detection of problems associated with tuberous sclerosis, thus leading to earlier treatment and better outcomes.

REFERENCES

Northrup H, Sing Au K. Tuberous sclerosis complex Bourneville disease. In: Pagon RA, Bird TC, Dolan CR, et al, eds. *GeneReviews*. Seattle: University of Washington; 2009.

Roach ES, Sparagana SP. Diagnosis of tuberous sclerosis complex. *J Child Neurol*. 2004;19:643–649.

Shields CL, Benevides R, Materin MA, et al. Optical coherence tomography of retinal astrocytic hamartoma in 15 cases. *Ophthalmology*. 2006;113:1553–1557.

Shields CL, Say EA, Fuller T, et al. Retinal astrocytic hamartoma arises in nerve fiber layer and shows "moth-eaten" optically empty spaces on optical coherence tomography. *Ophthalmology*. 2016;123:1809–1816.

Shields JA, Eagle Jr RC, Shields CL, et al. Aggressive retinal astrocytomas in 4 patients with tuberous sclerosis complex. *Arch Ophthalmol*. 2005;123:856–863.

Shields JA, Shields CL. *Atlas of Intraocular Tumors*. Philadelphia, PA: Lippincott Williams and Wilkins; 1999:269–286.

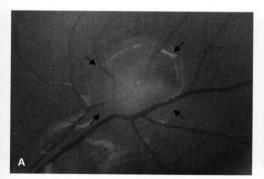
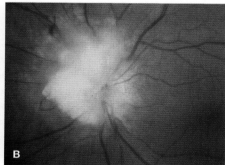

FIGURE 8-5. Astrocytic hamartoma. A. Small, ill-defined thickening of the nerve fiber layer. The *arrows* indicate the edge of the lesion. **B.** Large, opaque, calcified, sessile, whitish-yellow nodular mass ("mulberry lesion") at the optic nerve.

INCONTINENTIA PIGMENTI

Anuradha Ganesh and Alex V. Levin ■

Incontinentia pigmenti (IP), or Bloch-Sulzberger syndrome, is a rare X-linked dominant disorder of skin pigmentation that is accompanied by ocular, dental, and central nervous system (CNS) manifestations.

Epidemiology and Etiology

The incidence of incontinentia pigmenti is 1/40,000 live births. In most cases, incontinentia pigmenti is caused by mutations in the *NEMO* (NF-kappa-B essential modulator) gene at chromosome Xq28. As an X-linked dominant condition, it is usually lethal in males and thus is only seen in female infants. An affected male with Klinefelter syndrome (XXY) or genetic mosaicism may rarely survive. Incontinentia pigmenti refers to the histologic feature of "incontinence" of melanocytes in the basal layer of the epidermis of their pigment, which is then found in the superficial dermis.

History

Characteristic skin lesions are usually present at birth. Ophthalmic findings are noted in infancy or sometimes later in life. A pedigree may reveal a history of male fetus miscarriages.

Signs

The hallmark of ophthalmic involvement, present in over 40% of patients, is peripheral retinal capillary nonperfusion (Fig. 8-6). This avascular retina may be demarcated by an intervening peripheral ring of neovascularization or otherwise abnormal retinal vessels, reminiscent of the clinical findings in retinopathy of prematurity. Retinal ischemia leads to the arteriovenous anastomoses and neovascularization. The disease may resolve spontaneously, but 10% of infants develop retinal folds, traction, and rhegmatogenous retinal detachment with consequent visual impairment.

The ocular abnormalities are often asymmetric. Other eye findings are largely secondary and include strabismus in one-third of infants, cataracts, and retinal pigmentary changes with mottled, diffuse hypopigmentation, and foveal hypoplasia.

Skin findings include vesicular eruptions at birth that later evolve into desquamating erythematous lesions (Fig. 8-7A) followed by swirling hyperpigmentation (marble-cake appearance; Fig. 8-7B) and then scarring. Dental abnormalities occur in over 90% of affected individuals and include hypodontia, delayed eruption, and malformed, cone-shaped crowns. Associated CNS abnormalities include seizures, spastic paralysis, and mental retardation.

Differential Diagnosis

- Retinopathy of prematurity
- Familial exudative vitreoretinopathy
- Sickle cell disease (in older children)
- Other causes of infantile retinal nonattachment or detachment should also be considered.

Diagnostic Evaluation

The diagnosis of incontinentia pigmenti is based on clinical criteria (Table 8-2). Tests that may help in confirming the diagnosis include skin biopsy (although there is a wide differential diagnosis for the findings described earlier), neuroimaging (cerebral atrophy, agenesis of corpus callosum), fluorescein angiography (avascular peripheral retina, anomalous vessels in vascular-avascular junction), and genetic testing (for mutations in the *NEMO* gene). Careful skin, dental, and ocular examination of the patient's mother may be useful as variable expression.

Treatment and Prognosis

Patients with incontinentia pigmenti require careful retinal examination early in infancy to detect peripheral retinal nonperfusion. If present,

TABLE 8-2. Diagnostic Criteria for
Incontinentia Pigmenti

Major Criteria
Four stages of skin lesions from infancy to adulthood:
A. Linear vesicles and bullae of stage 1
B. Dark brown colored verrucous papules and plaques of stage 2
C. Light brown colored swirling hyperpigmentation of stage 3
D. White atrophic patches of stage 4

Minor Criteria
A. Teeth: hypodontia, anodontia, or microdontia
B. Hair: alopecia, wiry hair
C. Nails: mild ridging or pitting
D. Retina: peripheral neovascularization

The clinical diagnosis of incontinentia pigmenti can be made if at least one of the major criteria is present. The presence of minor criteria supports the clinical diagnosis; the complete absence of minor criteria should raise doubt regarding the diagnosis.
Adapted from Landy SJ, Donnai D. Incontinentia pigmenti (Bloch-Sulzberger syndrome). *J Med Genet.* 1993;30:53–59.

frequent follow-up is indicated to enable early detection of change that might suggest development of retinal neovascularization, vascular leakage, and traction. No treatment is indicated unless such changes develop, in which case laser photocoagulation is performed in an effort to prevent progression to retinal traction and detachment. One long-term follow-up study indicated a bimodal distribution of retinal detachments, with early childhood traction retinal detachments in some patients and later adult rhegmatogenous retinal detachments. Lifetime follow-up is needed. Genetic counseling is also highly recommended.

REFERENCES

Chen CJ, Han IC, Tian J, et al. Extended follow-up of treated and untreated retinopathy in incontinentia pigmenti: analysis of peripheral vascular changes and incidence of retinal detachment. *JAMA Ophthalmol.* 2015;133:542–548.

Holmstrom G, Thoren K. Ocular manifestations of incontinentia pigmenti. *Acta Ophthalmol Scand.* 2000;78:348–353.

Landy SJ, Donnai D. Incontinentia pigmenti (Bloch-Sulzberger syndrome). *J Med Genet.* 1993;30:53–59.

Scheuerle A, Ursini MV. Incontinentia pigmenti (Bloch-Sulzberger syndrome). In: Pagon RA, Bird TC, Dolan CR, Stephens K, eds. *GeneReviews.* Seattle, WA: University of Washington; 2010.

Smahi A, Courtois G, Vabres P, et al. Genomic rearrangement in NEMO impairs NF-kappaB activation and is a cause of incontinentia pigmenti. The International Incontinentia Pigmenti (IP) Consortium. *Nature.* 2000;405:466–472.

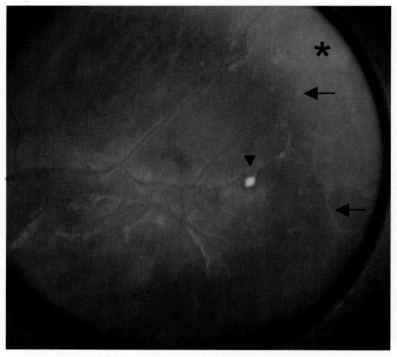

FIGURE 8-6. **Incontinentia Pigmenti (IP).** Fundus of a patient with IP showing peripheral retinal capillary nonperfusion (*asterisk*), arteriovenous anastomoses (*arrows*), and exudates (*arrowhead*).

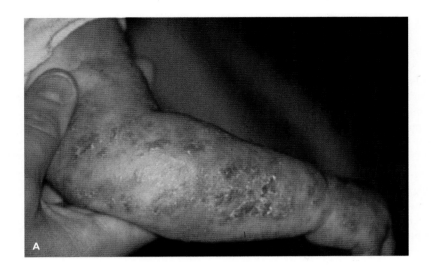

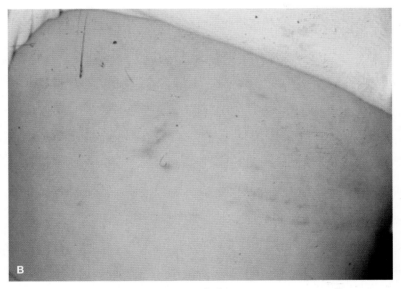

FIGURE 8-7. Skin findings in Incontinentia Pigmenti (IP). Vesicular and desquamating erythematous lesions in an infant with IP (**A**) and swirling hyperpigmentation ("marble-cake" appearance) (**B**).

COATS DISEASE

Barry N. Wasserman and Carol L. Shields ■

Coats disease is a nonhereditary condition characterized by unilateral retinal telangiectasia, exudation, and exudative retinal detachment that occurs most often in young patients.

Etiology

Coats disease is more common in males and generally occurs as a unilateral trait. The average age at onset is 2 to 8 years. Telangiectatic arterioles or venules lead to subretinal and intraretinal exudation of fluid and lipid, which eventually leads to exudative retinal detachment and vision loss. There is some evidence that Coats disease is related to a somatic mutation in the Norrie disease protein (*NDP*) gene or the frizzled 4 gene (*FZD4*).

Symptoms

The symptoms include painless vision loss, particularly when the disease occurs at an older age. Younger patients often present with strabismus or xanthocoria. Rarely, patients manifest neovascular glaucoma and a red, painful eye. In an analysis of 150 cases of Coats disease, the symptoms included decreased visual acuity (43%), strabismus (23%), xanthocoria (20%), pain (3%), heterochromia (1%), nystagmus (1%), and no symptoms (8%).

Signs

The findings in Coats disease include telangiectasia (100%), retinal exudation (99%), exudative retinal detachment (81%), retinal hemorrhage (13%), retinal macrocyst (11%), vasoproliferative tumor (6%), and neovascularization of disc (2%), retina (1%), and iris (8%). Anterior chamber cholesterolosis occurs in 3% of cases.

Differential Diagnosis

- Retinoblastoma
- Retinopathy of prematurity
- Retinal hemangioblastoma
- Retinal vasoproliferative tumor
- Sickle cell retinopathy
- Familial exudative vitreoretinopathy
- Toxocariasis
- Leukemia
- Persistent fetal vasculature (persistent hyperplastic primary vitreous)
- Radiation retinopathy
- Retinopathy of hypertensive crisis
- Cataract
- Coloboma

Diagnostic Evaluation

The diagnosis is established by recognition of the clinical features on ophthalmoscopy. Retinal telangiectatic vessels with fusiform and nodular vascular dilation and adjacent nonperfusion are found, classically in the temporal quadrant. Related intraretinal and subretinal exudation is noted and often retinal detachment is found (**Figs. 8-8** and **8-9**). Fluorescein angiography confirms these findings and additionally reveals vascular leakage and macular edema. The classification of Coats disease, proposed by Shields et al, is:

Stage 1: Retinal telangiectasia (T)

Stage 2: T + exudation (E)

Stage 3: T + E + subretinal fluid (F)

Stage 4: T + E + F + neovascular glaucoma (G)

Stage 5: T + E + F + G + phthisis bulbi

Treatment

Laser photocoagulation and cryotherapy are used to obliterate leaking vessels. The role of intravitreal antivascular endothelial growth factors is being explored. Pars plana vitrectomy with drainage of subretinal fluid and exudation is used for advanced cases.

Prognosis

Visual prognosis is often poor. In one analysis of 150 cases, poor visual acuity of 20/200 or worse was found in no patient with stage 1 disease, whereas 50% of stage 2, 70% of stage 3, and 100% of stages 4 and 5 show poor vision. The goal of treatment is stabilization of the eye with resolution of retinal detachment and exudation and prevention of neovascular glaucoma and loss of the eye. There are no systemic implications. However, patients with bilateral "Coats" disease should be evaluated for systemic syndromes.

REFERENCES

Morris B, Foot B, Mulvihill A. A population-based study of Coats disease in the United Kingdom I: epidemiology and clinical features at diagnosis. *Eye (Lond)*. 2010;24(12):1797–1801.

Mulvihill A, Morris B. A population-based study of Coats disease in the United Kingdom II: investigation, treatment, and outcomes. *Eye (Lond)*. 2010;4(12):1802–1807.

Shields JA, Shields CL Honavar S, Demirci H. Coats disease. Clinical variations and complications of Coats' disease in 150 cases. The 2000 Sanford Gifford Memorial Lecture. *Am J Ophthalmol*. 2001;131:561–571.

Shields JA, Shields CL, Honavar SG, et al. Classification and management of Coats disease. The 2000 Proctor lecture. *Am J Ophthalmol*. 2001;131:572–583.

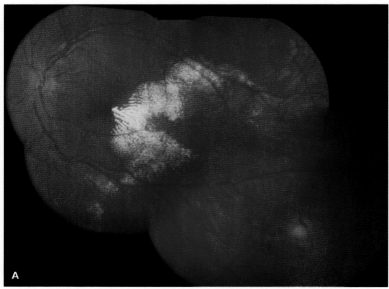

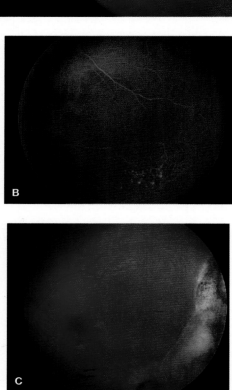

FIGURE 8-8. **Coats disease.** Coats disease (stage 2) with mild temporal macular exudation (**A**) from telangiectatic vessels (**B**) that showed resolution following therapy (**C**) with cryotherapy and laser photocoagulation, allowing for good visual acuity.

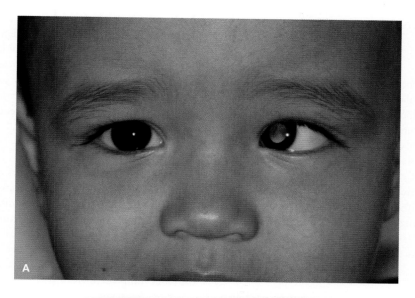

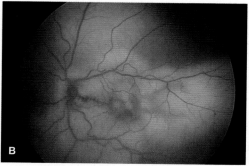

FIGURE 8-9. Coats disease. Coats disease (stage 3) with xanthocoria (**A**) from massive subretinal exudation (**B**) and leaking retinal telangiectasia (**C**).

RETINOBLASTOMA

Carol L. Shields ■

Retinoblastoma is the most common intraocular malignancy of children. It accounts for 4% of all childhood cancers. It is grouped into unilateral or bilateral involvement and subgrouped into sporadic or familial predisposition. This tumor manifests in young children, often those within the first year of life. Worldwide, it is estimated that there are approximately 7202 children per year with retinoblastoma distributed in Asia excluding Japan (4027), Africa (1792), Latin America/Caribbean (622), Europe (414), North America (258), Japan (59), and Oceania (21).

Etiology

Retinoblastoma occurs in approximately 1 in 15,000 live births. Children with bilateral retinoblastoma are typically diagnosed around 12 months and those with unilateral retinoblastoma around 18 months. There is no race or gender predilection. Approximately 2/3 of all cases are unilateral and 1/3 are bilateral.

Retinoblastoma results from mutation of the *Rb* gene located on chromosome 13q14. In 1971, Knudson's "two-hit" hypothesis for the development of retinoblastoma was proposed. In 1980, research confirmed that both alleles of retinoblastoma gene (*RB1*) at chromosome 13q14 locus were mutated in retinoblastoma. Currently, there are arguments that genomic instability and aneuploidy are likely responsible for the genesis of *Rb*.

Bilateral and familial retinoblastomas arise from germ line mutation in the retinoblastoma gene whereas unilateral disease is more often a result of somatic mutation but can result from germ line mutation in 15% of cases. Germ line mutation retinoblastoma tends to be multifocal and can be associated with systemic cancers such as pinealoblastoma and remote cancers. A small subset of retinoblastoma patients display the 13q syndrome which occurs from the mutation on chromosome 13 and involves features of microcephaly, broad nasal bridge, hypertelorism, microphthalmos, epicanthus, ptosis, micrognathia, short neck, low-set ears, facial asymmetry, anogenital malformations, hypoplastic thumbs and toes, and mental and psychomotor retardation.

Symptoms

Retinoblastoma most often presents quietly with the painless development of leukocoria or strabismus (**Fig. 8-10**). It is most often discovered by the parents or grandparents more so than pediatricians. Occasionally, the child might have pain from secondary glaucoma that manifests in about 17% of patients. Rarely does the child complain of vision loss.

Signs

The anterior segment classically displays leukocoria, and this feature is more prominent relative to tumor size. Neovascularization of the iris is occasionally found.

Fundoscopically, retinoblastoma appears as a solid, yellow-white tumor within the retina. It can appear with different growth patterns such as intraretinal, subretinal (exophytic), vitreal (endophytic), and flat (diffuse). Small tumors appear intraretinal with a slightly dilated artery and vein. As the tumor enlarges, the vessels dilate and become slightly tortuous. Calcification can develop within the mass. Subretinal fluid, subretinal seeds, and vitreous seeds then develop. Occasionally, seeds can extend into the anterior chamber producing a neoplastic pseudohypopyon. Advanced tumors lead to neovascularization of the iris with glaucoma, retinal neovascularization with vitreous hemorrhage, and invasion into the optic nerve and choroid.

Differential Diagnosis

● Retinal detachment from retinoblastoma can simulate:

   ■ Coats disease

- Persistent hyperplastic primary vitreous (persistent fetal vasculature)
- Toxocariasis
- Retinal astrocytic hamartoma
- Retinal astrocytoma
- Combined hamartoma of the retina and RPE
- Retinal detachment
- Familial exudative vitreoretinopathy
- Retinopathy of prematurity
- Incontinentia pigmenti
- Vitreous seeding from retinoblastoma can simulate:
  - Intraocular inflammation
  - Endophthalmitis
  - Vitreous hemorrhage
  - Leukemic infiltration
- Leukocoria from retinoblastoma can simulate:
  - Cataract
  - Glaucoma

Diagnostic Evaluation

The diagnosis of retinoblastoma is established in the office setting using indirect ophthalmoscopy in the hands of an experienced examiner. Examination under anesthesia is reserved for detailed analysis of each eye, confirmation with diagnostic tests, and therapy. The tumor is confirmed on ultrasonography, showing it as a calcified dome-shaped mass. Fluorescein angiography will show intrinsic luxurious vascularity. OCT will show subretinal fluid in cooperative children. Computed tomography (CT) will confirm the calcification within the mass, but most clinicians prefer magnetic resonance imaging (MRI) to CT because there is no radiation exposure with the former. MRI will show the enhancing intraocular mass and can be used to image the orbit and the brain, evaluating for optic nerve invasion and pinealoblastoma. Fine-needle aspiration biopsy should be avoided.

Each affected eye is classified according to the International Classification of Retinoblastoma (ICRB) (**Fig. 8-11**):

- Group A: retinoblastoma ≤3 mm
- Group B: retinoblastoma >3 mm or in the macula or with clear subretinal the fluid
- Group C: retinoblastoma with subretinal or vitreous seeds ≤3 mm from th e tumor
- Group D: retinoblastoma with subretinal or vitreous seeds >3 mm from tumor
- Group E: extensive retinoblastoma fill >50% globe or with hemorrhage or iris neovascularization

Treatment

Retinoblastoma management is complex and depends on many issues including tumor laterality, macular involvement, tumor size, vitreous or subretinal seeding, relationship of the tumor to surrounding tissues including the optic disc, choroid, iris, sclera, and orbit, general patient age and health, and the family wishes. Laser photocoagulation, cryotherapy, thermotherapy, and plaque radiotherapy remain vitally important in the management of selective retinoblastoma. Enucleation, intravenous chemoreduction, intra-arterial chemotherapy, and external beam radiotherapy are used for more advanced retinoblastoma. External beam radiotherapy is usually reserved for last alternative treatment because of its numerous side effects and risks for late-onset cancers in germ line mutation children.

Enucleation is used for advanced eyes, particularly unilateral tumors. Following enucleation, the eye should be evaluated pathologically for high-risk features.

Systemic intravenous chemoreduction is used for bilateral cases in which there are multiple tumors and often seeding (**Fig. 8-12**). Groups A, B, and C show >90% success with chemoreduction and group D shows about 50% success. Group E eyes are often enucleated.

Intra-arterial chemotherapy is showing promise as a primary treatment for retinoblastoma and after failure of other methods. In our preliminary experience, we have had 100% tumor control for groups C and D retinoblastoma and 33% control for group E (Fig. 8-13). Groups A and B retinoblastoma are not offered intra-arterial chemotherapy yet as there are potentially profound risks such as cerebrovascular accident and ophthalmic artery obstruction.

In rare instances, retinoblastoma can undergo spontaneous regression and show clinical features of complete tumor resolution without therapeutic intervention. Occasionally, this can lead to phthisis bulbi.

Prognosis

Retinoblastoma is a highly malignant tumor with nearly 100% mortality if left untreated. In developed nations, most children present before high-risk features are found; thus, good prognosis with life-saving measures is achieved. In an analysis of retinoblastoma worldwide, mortality paralleled the development of the nation.

There are histopathologic factors that predict metastatic disease, including optic nerve invasion beyond the lamina cribrosa, massive choroidal invasion > 3 mm, scleral invasion, orbital invasion, and anterior chamber invasion. Some globes enucleated with retinoblastoma have high-risk features such as retrolaminar optic nerve invasion or massive uveal invasion of more than 3 mm. Patients with these features should receive additional chemotherapy.

Children with germinal retinoblastoma have an increased risk of developing other primary malignancies over the course of their lifetimes. These tumors include principally intracranial retinoblastoma, osteogenic sarcoma of the long bones, and sarcoma of soft tissues. The risk is estimated to be 30% by age 30, and the use of external beam radiotherapy can increase the risk in the field of irradiation.

REFERENCES

Eagle RC Jr. High-risk features and tumor differentiation in retinoblastoma: a retrospective histopathologic study. *Arch Pathol Lab Med.* 2009;133:1203–1209.

Kivela T. The epidemiological challenge of the most frequent eye cancer: retinoblastoma, an issue of birth and death. *Br J Ophthalmol.* 2009;93:1129–1131.

Shields CL, Shields JA. Basic understanding of current classification and management of retinoblastoma. *Curr Opin Ophthalmol.* 2006;17:228–234.

Shields CL, Shields JA. Retinoblastoma management: advances in enucleation, intravenous chemoreduction, and intra-arterial chemotherapy. *Curr Opin Ophthalmol.* 2010;21:203–212.

Shields JA, Shields CL. Retinoblastoma. In: Shields JA, Shields CL. *Atlas of Intraocular Tumors.* Philadelphia, PA: Lippincott Williams Wilkins; 2008:293–365.

Wong FL, Boice JD Jr, Abramson DH, et al. Cancer incidence after retinoblastoma. Radiation dose and sarcoma risk. *JAMA.* 1997;278:1262–1267.

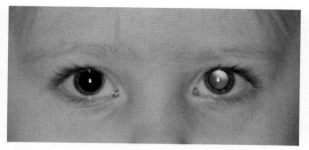

FIGURE 8-10. **Retinoblastoma.** Leukocoria (left eye) from retinoblastoma.

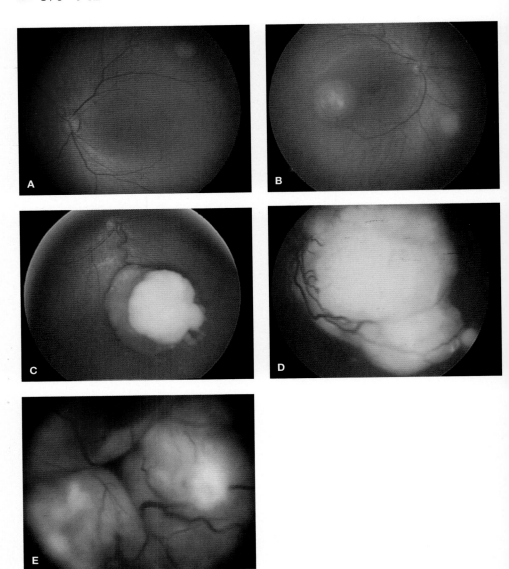

FIGURE 8-11. Retinoblastoma. Examples of the international classification of retinoblastoma into groups **A, B, C, D,** and **E.**

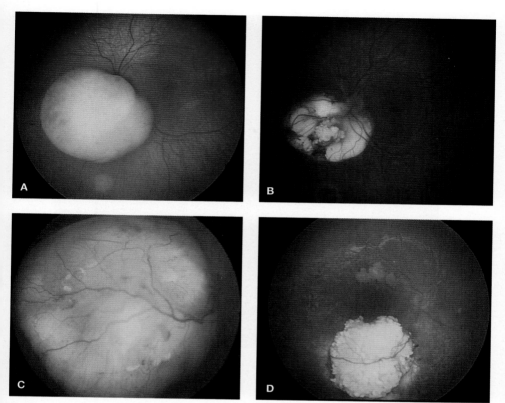

FIGURE 8-12. Retinoblastoma. Response of retinoblastoma to intravenous chemoreduction in two cases before therapy (**A** and **C**) and after therapy (**B** and **D**).

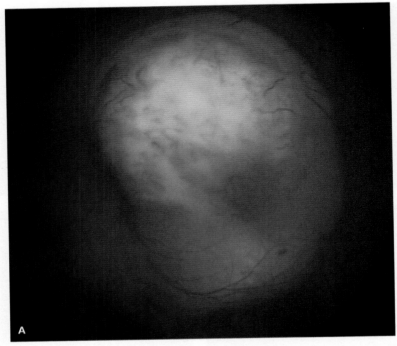

FIGURE 8-13. Retinoblastoma. Response of retinoblastoma to intra-arterial chemotherapy showing before therapy (**A**) and after therapy (**B**).

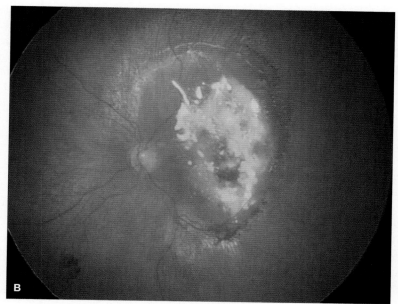

FIGURE 8-13. (*Continued*)

CONGENITAL HYPERTROPHY OF THE RETINAL PIGMENT EPITHELIUM

Anuradha Ganesh and Alex V. Levin ■

Congenital hypertrophy of the retinal pigment epithelium (CHRPE) is a benign, asymptomatic condition, consisting of one or more well-demarcated, pigmented, flat, nonmitotic lesions at the level of the RPE.

Epidemiology and Etiology

Solitary CHRPE occurs in approximately 1/60 in the general population. No racial predilection has been reported. Histopathologically, the lesion consists of a focal area in which the RPE cells are taller and more densely packed with melanosomes. The individual melanosomes are larger and more spherical as compared with those of the normal RPE. The associated depigmented lacunae, halos, or "tails" correspond to areas where the melanosomes are sparse.

History

Patients are usually asymptomatic. Often the disorder is noted as an incidental finding during ophthalmoscopy.

Signs

CHRPE may take one of two forms:

● Solitary: This is the most common form. It is characteristically a unilateral, deeply pigmented, flat, circular lesion, with a well-circumscribed margin. These may be pinpoint or two or three disc diameters in size. The lesion may be solid black with a marginal halo of hypopigmentation. Depigmented lacunae may be seen within the lesion.

● Multiple: Multifocal CHRPE lesions are seen in over 80% of patients with familial adenomatous polyposis (FAP) or Gardner syndrome, a familial condition of colonic polyps and extraintestinal osteomas and fibromas with uniform progression to colonic cancer if not treated. The lesions are bilateral, multiple, scattered, and more often have a "cometoid" configuration with a hypopigmented tail on the side of the lesion closer to the macula (**Fig. 8-14**).

Differential Diagnosis

● Choroidal melanoma

● Choroidal nevus

● Combined hamartoma of the retina and RPE

● Reactive hyperplasia of the RPE (e.g., posttraumatic)

● Bear tracks

● Chorioretinal scars (e.g., toxoplasmosis, congenital varicella)

Diagnostic Evaluation

The characteristic appearance of CHRPE should enable the clinician to make the diagnosis and differentiate it from other lesions. Fluorescein angiography reveals hypofluorescence throughout all phases of the angiogram, except in the region of the haloes and lacunae, which show transmission hyperfluorescence. The lesions are not associated with subretinal fluid or orange pigment. Enhanced depth imaging OCT reveals flat lesions with irregular RPE and absent RPE in the lacunae. There may be loss of outer nuclear layer and retinal photoreceptors, and subretinal clefts.

Treatment and Prognosis

Although overlying photoreceptor loss and alterations of the RPE may lead to VF defects, CHRPEs are usually benign and asymptomatic and do not affect visual acuity or visual field. Over time, subtle enlargement of the lesions and development of an elevated nodule representing adenoma or adenocarcinoma has rarely been reported. Hence, they should be observed periodically for growth. Patients with bilateral or multiple unilateral lesions suggestive of those seen in FAP or Gardner syndrome should be referred for periodic colonoscopy usually beginning at 7 or 8 years of age.

REFERENCES

Fung AT, Pellegrini M, Shields CL. Congenital hypertrophy of the retinal pigment epithelium: enhanced-depth imaging optical coherence tomography in 18 cases. *Ophthalmology.* 2014;121:251–256.

Shields JA, Eagle RC Jr, Shields CL, et al. Malignant transformation of congenital hypertrophy of the retinal pigment epithelium. *Ophthalmology.* 2009;116:2213–2216.

Shields JA, Shields CL. Tumors and related lesions of the pigment epithelium. In: Shields JA, Shields CL, eds. *Intraocular Tumors. A Text and Atlas.* Philadelphia, PA: WB Saunders; 1992:437–460.

Traboulsi EI, Maumenee IH, Krush AJ, et al. Congenital hypertrophy of the retinal pigment epithelium predicts colorectal polyposis in Gardner's syndrome. *Arch Ophthalmol.* 1990;108:525–526.

Traboulsi EI. Ocular manifestations of familial adenomatous polyposis (Gardner syndrome). *Ophthalmol Clin North Am.* 2005;18:163–166.

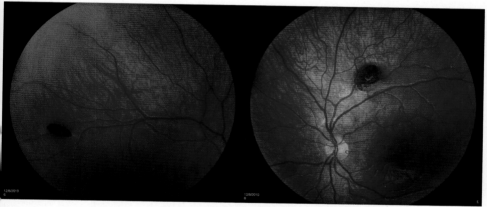

FIGURE 8-14. Congenital hypertrophy of the retinal pigment epithelium. Fundus photograph both retinas shows bilateral hyperpigmented retinal lesions in a patient with Gardner syndrome. The lesion in the right eye has a "cometoid" appearance with a hypopigmented tail on the side of the lesion closer to the macula. The lesions in both eyes show a marginal halo of depigmentation.

FAMILIAL EXUDATIVE VITREORETINOPATHY

Anuradha Ganesh and Alex V. Levin ■

Familial exudative vitreoretinopathy (FEVR) is a hereditary vitreoretinal disorder characterized by failure of peripheral retinal vascularization and resulting in secondary complications such as neovascularization, retinal folds, traction, and detachment.

Epidemiology and Etiology

FEVR is a rare disorder. The prevalence has not been calculated. Ninety percent of affected individuals may be asymptomatic. FEVR is genetically heterogeneous and is associated with mutations in the Frizzled-4 (*FZD4*; autosomal dominant FEVR), *LRP5* (autosomal dominant and recessive FEVR), *NDP* (X-linked recessive FEVR), and *TSPAN12* (autosomal dominant FEVR) genes. Autosomal dominant inheritance is the most common mode of inheritance.

History

The clinical appearance of FEVR varies considerably, even within families, with severely affected patients often registered as blind during infancy and mildly affected patients having few or no visual problems. Infants may present with strabismus or leukocoria due to retinal detachment. There is no association with prematurity or oxygen exposure.

Signs

Infants born with FEVR are otherwise healthy. Ophthalmic findings are frequently asymmetric and highly variable. The classic finding in FEVR is peripheral retinal capillary nonperfusion (Fig. 8-15). Usually, the avascular zone is confined to the temporal periphery, but it may extend for 360 degrees. The disease may not progress further or may lead to peripheral neovascularization at the border of posterior vascularized and anterior avascular retina (Fig. 8-16). Retinal fold, peripheral fibrovascular mass, vitreous hemorrhage, and progression to even more severe changes such as tractional, exudative, and even rhegmatogenous retinal detachment may occur. Intraretinal and subretinal exudation may be associated. In severe cases with retinal detachment, there may be cataract, band keratopathy, neovascular glaucoma, and/or phthisis. Asymptomatic individuals may manifest regions of peripheral avascularity with abnormal vascular anastomoses visible clinically or only on intravenous fluorescein angiography.

Differential Diagnosis

- Retinopathy of prematurity
- Incontinentia pigmenti
- Coats disease
- Persistent fetal vasculature
- Sickle cell retinopathy
- Other causes of infantile retinal nonattachment or detachment

Diagnostic Evaluation

The diagnosis of FEVR is based on a family history compatible with autosomal dominant, autosomal recessive, or X-linked recessive inheritance and bilateral peripheral retinal avascularity. If FEVR is suspected, examination of the peripheral retina of asymptomatic family members may also reveal findings consistent with the diagnosis. Tests that may help in confirming the diagnosis include fluorescein angiography (abrupt cessation of peripheral retinal capillary network and possible abnormal vasculature) and genetic testing. SD-OCT may reveal a broad spectrum of microstructural findings including dysgenic posterior hyaloid, cystoid macular edema, and both inner and outer retinal abnormalities.

Treatment and Prognosis

Laser photocoagulation to the peripheral avascular retina and neovascularization may prevent progression of fibrovascular complications. The value of prophylactic treatment is controversial and most authors suggest treatment only if neovascularization is present. Prevention of retinal detachment is far more effective than treatment once detachment occurs. FEVR is a lifelong disease, and events like neovascularization, retinal detachments, and vitreous hemorrhage may occur at any age. Perinatal screening, continued for several years, is advisable in at-risk individuals.

REFERENCES

Robitaille JM, Zheng B, Wallace K, et al. The role of Frizzled-4 mutations in familial exudative vitreoretinopathy and Coats disease. *Br J Ophthalmol.* 2011;95(4):574–579.

Shukla D, Singh J, Sudheer G, et al. Familial exudative vitreoretinopathy (FEVR). Clinical profile and management. *Indian J Ophthalmol.* 2003;51:323–328.

Toomes C, Downey L. Familial exudative vitreoretinopathy, autosomal dominant. In: Pagon RA, Bird TC, Dolan CR, Stephens K, ed. *GeneReviews.* Seattle: University of Washington; 2008.

Yonekawa Y, Thomas BJ, Drenser KA, et al. Familial exudative vitreoretinopathy: spectral-domain optical coherence tomography of the vitreoretinal interface, retina, and choroid. *Ophthalmology.* 2015;122:2270–2277.

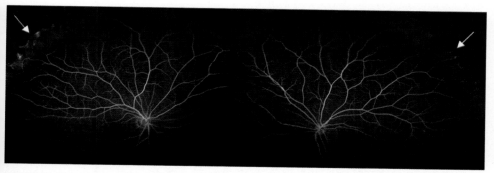

FIGURE 8-15. Familial exudative vitreoretinopathy. Fundus fluorescein angiogram clearly demonstrates bilateral peripheral retinal capillary nonperfusion and leakage (*arrows*).

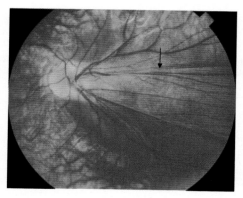

FIGURE 8-16. Familial exudative vitreoretinopathy. Retinal tractional fold (*arrow*) causing straightening of vessels at the disc.

PERSISTENT FETAL VASCULATURE

Alok S. Bansal ■

Persistent fetal vasculature (PFV), formerly referred to as persistent hyperplastic primary vitreous (PHPV), is a developmental malformation of the eye that results from failure of regression of the primary vitreal hyaloidal vessels and other associated vessels in the tunica vasculosa lentis and/or iris.

PFV is most often unilateral and nonheritable. When bilateral (10%), there is more often systemic associations and the potential for a genetic basis (**Table 8-3**).

Signs

There are many forms of PFV, ranging in a spectrum from anterior findings to posterior findings. Isolated anterior PFV (**Fig. 8-17A**) is characterized by a retrolental vascularized membrane, variable degree of cataract, drawn-in ciliary processes (**Fig. 8-17B**), traction on the peripheral retina due to a membranous transformation of the anterior vitreous face, shallow anterior chamber, poor pupil dilation, and microphthalmos. Congenital fibrovascular pupillary membranes may be an isolated variant of anterior PFV. The more severe posterior PFV is characterized by a stalk of tissue extending from the optic nerve to the retrolental area, a retinal fold with or without tractional retinal detachment (**Fig. 8-17C**), macular pigmentary disruption, and variable degrees of optic nerve dysplasia. The lens can be clear in isolated posterior PFV.

Differential Diagnosis

- Norrie disease
- Coats disease
- Toxocariasis
- Retinopathy of prematurity
- FEVR
- Incontinentia pigmenti
- Retinal dysplasia
- Retinal detachment (overt or covert trauma)

Diagnostic Evaluation

The diagnosis of PFV can be made with careful ophthalmoscopic exam. Depending on the age of the child, an exam under anesthesia may be considered. If significant media opacity precludes a view of the fundus, B-scan ultrasonography may demonstrate a stalk or retinal detachment. Careful examination of the iris may reveal anterior signs of persistent vasculature.

TABLE 8-3. Systemic and Genetic Basis of Ocular Disorders

Syndrome	Inheritance	Chromosome	Gene	Function
Wagner	AD	5q14.3	CSPG2	Binds to hyaluronan in vitreous
Knobloch	AR	21q22.3	COL18A1	Cleaves to endostatin
PFV	AR	10q11-21	Not known	
PFV	XLR	Xp11.4	NDP	Signaling pathways for morphogenesis
ASMD	AD	10q22.3-25	PITX3	Regulates ocular morphogenesis

AD, autosomal dominant; AR, autosomal recessive; ASMD, anterior segment mesenchymal dysgenesis; COL18A1, collagen type 18 alpha 1; CSPG, chondroitin sulfate proteoglycan; NDP, Norrie disease pseudoglioma; PFV, persistent fetal vasculature; PITX3, paired like homeodomain 3; XLR, X-linked recessive.

Treatment

The goals of management include clearing the media opacity in order to allow visual development and prevent complications of untreated PFV such as glaucoma and retinal detachment. Either anterior limbal or pars plana approaches to lensectomy, membranectomy, and vitrectomy may be employed. Aggressive amblyopia treatment with aphakic contact lenses are required to achieve optimum vision. The prognosis for pure anterior PFV is better than posterior PFV.

REFERENCES

Goldberg MF. Persistent fetal vasculature (PFV): an integrated interpretation of signs and symptoms associated with persistent hyperplastic primary vitreous (PHPV). LIV Edward Jackson Memorial Lecture. *Am J Ophthalmol.* 1997;124(5):587–626.

Lambert SR, Buckley EG, Lenhart PD, et al. Congenital fibrovascular pupillary membranes: clinical and histopathologic findings. *Ophthalmology.* 2012;199:634–641.

Pollard, ZF. Persistent hyperplastic primary vitreous: diagnosis, treatment, and results. *Trans Am Ophthalmol Soc.* 1997;95:487–549.

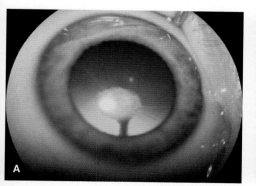

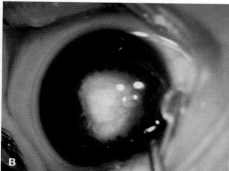

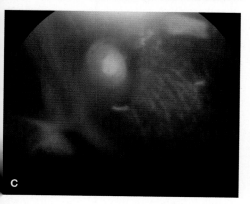

FIGURE 8-17. Persistent fetal vasculature (PFV). **A.** The retrolental stalk is due to failure of regression of the primary vitreal hyaloidal vessels. **B.** PFV demonstrating a vascularized retrolental membrane, cataract, and drawn-in ciliary processes. **C.** PFV demonstrating a retinal fold with an associated tractional retinal detachment.

JUVENILE RETINOSCHISIS

Barry N. Wasserman ■

Etiology

An X-linked inherited disease, juvenile retinoschisis is the most common cause of macular degeneration in young males. Mutation of the *XLRS1* gene results in retinal dysfunction due to splitting of the retinal layers and the characteristic inner retinal layer schisis and stellate maculopathy.

Symptoms

Patients may present with mildly reduced vision that may deteriorate to less than 20/400, though one study suggested no significant disease progression in children over an average of 12 years of follow-up. Visual loss is caused by foveal schisis or retinal detachment.

Signs

Fundus examination reveals foveal schisis in a stellate pattern. In approximately 50% of patients, peripheral retinoschisis of the nerve fiber layer occurs with inner layer holes and possible progression to full-thickness retinal detachment. Whitish dots or patches in the retinal midperiphery and periphery (snowflakes) may be seen and are thought to represent abnormal Müller cell footplates. Pigmented demarcation lines indicate prior full-thickness detachment. Spontaneous vitreous hemorrhage results from vessels bridging the inner retinal layer holes.

Differential Diagnosis

- Nicotinic acid maculopathy
- Rhegmatogenous retinal detachment
- Goldmann–Favre disease
- Wagner vitreoretinal dystrophy and other vitreoretinopathies
- Cystoid macular edema
- Norrie disease

Diagnostic Evaluation

Characteristic family history of affected males with intervening unaffected female carriers. Fundus examination reveals stellate appearance in fovea, which resembles cystoid macular edema (Fig. 8-18). Fluorescein angiography does not show leakage. Retinal pigment epithelial pigmentary changes and vitreous veils are seen. Optical coherence tomography may demonstrate schisis extending into the retinal periphery (Fig. 8-19). One study using SD-OCT demonstrated increased inner foveal thickness and decreased perifoveal inner retinal thickness correlating with worse visual acuity. Electroretinogram reveals diminished B-wave amplitudes, but electrooculogram is normal.

Treatment

Genetic counseling is recommended for families with X-linked juvenile retinoschisis. Some patients with cystoid macular changes have shown improvement in visual acuity and OCT finding when treated with topical or oral carbonic anhydrase inhibitors. Prophylactic laser photocoagulation is not recommended and can lead to retinal detachment. Surgery utilizing scleral buckling and pars plana vitrectomy can be performed for vitreous hemorrhage and retinal detachment.

Prognosis

Some patients maintain good vision into adulthood, but visual acuity commonly deteriorates particularly when peripheral retinal schisis is present.

REFERENCES

Andreoli MT, Lim JI. Optical coherence tomography retinal thickness and volume measurements in X-linked retinoschisis. *Am J Ophthalmol.* 2014;158:567–573.

Apushkin MA, Fishman GA. Use of dorzolamide for patients with X-linked retinoschisis. *Retina.* 2006;26:741–745.

Goodwin P. Hereditary retinal disease. *Curr Opin Ophthalmol.* 2008;19:255–262.

Kjellström S, Vijayasarathy C, Ponjavic V, et al. Long-term 12 year follow-up of X-linked congenital retinoschisis. *Ophthalmic Genet.* 2010;31(3):114–125.

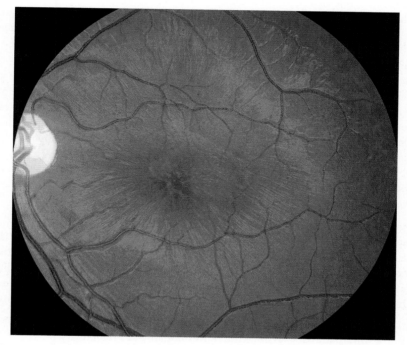

FIGURE 8-18. Juvenile X-linked retinoschisis. Juvenile X-linked retinoschisis with cystic appearance in the macula.

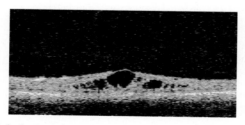

FIGURE 8-19. Juvenile X-linked retinoschisis. Optical coherence tomography of macula demonstrating schisis cavities.

RETINOPATHY OF PREMATURITY

Anuradha Ganesh and Barry N. Wasserman ■

Retinopathy of prematurity (ROP) is a proliferative retinopathy of premature, low-birth-weight infants.

Epidemiology and Etiology

Each year, ROP is believed to affect an estimated 14,000 to 16,000 premature, low-birth-weight infants in the United States. The majority of infants who develop ROP undergo spontaneous regression (85%). The rest will develop severe ROP requiring treatment, and 6% to 7% of infants will become legally blind despite treatment. Infants born before 32 weeks of gestation or those with a birth weight of less than 1500 g who have received oxygen therapy are at risk.

In preterm infants, retinal vascular development is incomplete. Instead of continued progression from the optic nerve head anteriorly along the plane of retina, vascular migration ceases, leading to an area of avascular retina. The extent of avascular retina depends mainly on the degree of prematurity at birth. The resultant hypoxia stimulates production of substances such as vascular endothelial growth factor (VEGF) which trigger neovascularization, known as extraretinal fibrovascular proliferation (ERFP), off the surface of the retina. ERFP may lead to hemorrhage and contraction with resultant retinal detachment. In many cases, the retinopathy abnormalities spontaneously regress without treatment.

History

Infants are considered high risk and are screened for ROP if birth weight is less than 1500 g or gestational age is 32 weeks or less. Selected infants with an unstable clinical course, including those requiring cardiorespiratory support, with a birth weight between 1500 and 2000 g, or gestational age of more than 32 weeks, may also be screened at the discretion of the neonatologist.

Signs

The International Classification of ROP (ICROP) categorizes ROP by location, called the Zone, or by severity, called the Stage. In addition, the presence or absence of *plus disease* is evaluated (**Table 8-4, Fig. 8-20**). An eye has plus disease

TABLE 8-4. International Classification of Retinopathy of Prematurity

Location	
Zone I	Posterior circle of retina centered on the optic nerve with a radius of twice the disc-fovea distance
Zone II	Circular area of retina from the edge of Zone I to the nasal ora serrata
Zone III	Remaining temporal crescent of retina
Extent	
Number of clock hours or 30-degree sectors involved	
Severity	
Stage 1	Demarcation line at the junction of posterior vascularized and anterior avascular retina
Stage 2	Ridge (demarcation line with volume)
Stage 3	Ridge with extraretinal fibrovascular proliferation
Stage 4	Subtotal retinal detachment
Stage 4A	Extrafoveal
Stage 4B	Fovea is detached
Stage 5	Total retinal detachment with funnel

Reprinted with permission from International Committee for the Classification of Retinopathy of Prematurity. The International Classification of Retinopathy of Prematurity revisited [review]. *Arch Ophthalmol.* 2005;123(7):991–999.

when there are at least two quadrants of dilatation of veins and tortuosity of arterioles in the posterior pole (**Fig. 8-20C**). Iris engorgement, pupillary rigidity, vitreous haze, or retinal hemorrhages are often seen in plus disease. Plus disease denotes increased severity. *Pre-plus disease* refers to more mild posterior pole vascular dilation and tortuosity, that is insufficient for diagnosis of plus disease.

"Popcorn" lesions are named so because of their similarity to kernels of white fluffy popcorn floating above the developed retina. They represent buds of vascular proliferation behind the ridge or demarcation line. Popcorn is only significant when part of active ERFP. Vitreous hemorrhage and preretinal hemorrhage can occasionally be seen in eyes with severe ERFP.

In acute posterior ROP (AP-ROP), vascularization is only present in Zone I and there is plus disease. This subtype of ROP previously termed "rush" disease is associated with an aggressive course and a risk for rapid progression into stage 4 or 5.

After treatment of ROP, most will regress by a process of involution or cicatrization, often yielding good visual acuity. This may be accompanied by a broad range of sequelae such as failure of peripheral retinal vascularization, abnormal branching of retinal vessels, retinal pigmentary changes, vitreoretinal interface changes, retinal folds, and distortion and ectopia of the macula.

The characteristic findings of ROP are present in the setting of infants born prematurely, of low birth weight with a history of oxygen exposure and other disorders associated with prematurity such as sepsis, intraventricular hemorrhage, anemia, and feeding difficulties.

Differential Diagnosis

Differential diagnosis depends on the stage of the disease.

- In less severe ROP, conditions that cause peripheral retinal vascular changes and retinal dragging should be considered:
  - Incontinentia pigmenti
  - FEVR
  - PFV
  - Other causes of infantile retinal nonattachment or detachment
- In advanced cicatricial ROP, the differential diagnosis is consistent with retinal detachment or leukocoria:
  - Retinoblastoma
  - Cataract
  - Coats disease
  - Toxocariasis

Diagnostic Evaluation

Careful examination of neonates with indirect ophthalmoscopy in the intensive care nursery or at discharge is recommended between 4 and 6 weeks of chronologic (postnatal) age or, alternatively, within the 31st to 33rd week of postconceptional or postmenstrual age (gestational age at birth plus chronologic age), whichever is later. Digital imaging is an useful adjunct during fundus examinations.

Treatment and Prognosis

The purpose of screening for ROP is to identify infants with advanced ROP who would progress to retinal detachment unless treated. Older treatment criteria utilized the term 'threshold', but this has now been replaced by 'Type 1 and Type 2.' *"Prethreshold" disease* is defined as any Zone I-stage of ROP or Zone II-stage 2 + ROP/stage 3 ROP/stage 3 + ROP but less extensive than threshold disease. The early treatment for ROP (ET-ROP) study divided prethreshold eyes into two groups (**Table 8-5**) and recommended that peripheral retinal ablation be applied to any eye with type 1 prethreshold ROP.

Peripheral retinal ablation of the anterior avascular zone may be performed with cryotherapy or laser photocoagulation. The latter, delivered with an indirect ophthalmoscope, has replaced cryotherapy for threshold ROP (**Fig. 8-21**). Better visual outcomes have been achieved with laser treatment. More advanced stages of ROP (stages 4 and 5) require scleral buckling or vitrectomy, or both. The prognosis

TABLE 8-5. Early Treatment of ROP
Prethreshold Types

Type I
Zone I: any stage ROP with plus disease
Zone I: stage 3 ROP without plus disease
Zone II: stage 2 or 3 ROP with plus disease

Type II
Zone I: stage 1 or 2 ROP without plus disease
Zone II: stage 3 ROP without plus disease

ROP, retinopathy of prematurity.
Reprinted with permission from Vander JF, McNamara
JA, Tasman W, et al. Revised indications for early
treatment of retinopathy of prematurity. *Arch Ophthalmol.*
2005;123:406–407.

for visual recovery after retinal detachment
remains poor.

Despite appropriate screening and timing of
intervention, ROP in some babies continues to
progress. This has led to research into newer and
more effective modalities of therapy. Ongoing
studies evaluating the efficacy and safety of intravitreal injections of anti-VEGF drugs for ROP
suggest this therapeutic modality may produce
similar or better outcomes than laser photocoagulation. However, use of anti-VEGF drugs has been
associated with late recurrence of the ROP, and
vigilant follow-up every 1 to 2 weeks for up to 55
weeks may be indicated. These medications escape
the eye and may lead to temporary impairment
of systemic vasculature development. One study

recommended caution after an increased incidence
of developmental delay was noted in children
treated with anti-VEGF for ROP.

REFERENCES
Davitt BV, Wallace DK. Plus disease. *Surv Ophthalmol.*
2009;54:663–670.
Kemper AR, Wallace DK, Quinn GE. Systematic review of
digital imaging screening strategies for retinopathy of
prematurity. *Pediatrics.* 2008;122:825–830.
Mintz-Hittner HA, Geloneck MM, Chuang AZ. Clinical
management of recurrent retinopathy of prematurity after
intravitreal bevacizumab monotherapy. *Ophthalmology.*
2016;123:1845–1855.
Mintz-Hittner HA, Kuffel RR Jr. Intravitreal injection of
bevacizumab (avastin) for treatment of stage 3 retinopathy of prematurity in zone I or posterior zone II. *Retina.*
2008;28:831–838.
Morin J, Luu TM, Superstein R, et al; Canadian Neonatal
Network and the Canadian Neonatal Follow-Up Network
Investigators. Neurodevelopmental outcomes following
bevacizumab injections for retinopathy of prematurity.
Pediatrics. 2016;137:e20153218.
Patel JR, Ranjan SS, Wasserman BN. Antivascular
endothelial growth factor in the treatment of ret-
inopathy of prematurity. *Curr Opin Ophthalmol.*
2016;27:387–392.
Reynolds JD. Retinopathy of prematurity. *Int Ophthalmol
Clin.* 2010;50:1–13.
Section on Ophthalmology American Academy of Pediat-
rics; American Academy of Ophthalmology; American
Association for Pediatric Ophthalmology and Strabismus.
Screening examination of premature infants for retinop-
athy of prematurity. *Pediatrics.* 2006;117(2):572–576.
Vander JF, McNamara JA, Tasman W, et al. Revised indica-
tions for early treatment of retinopathy of prematurity.
Arch Ophthalmol. 2005;123:406–407.

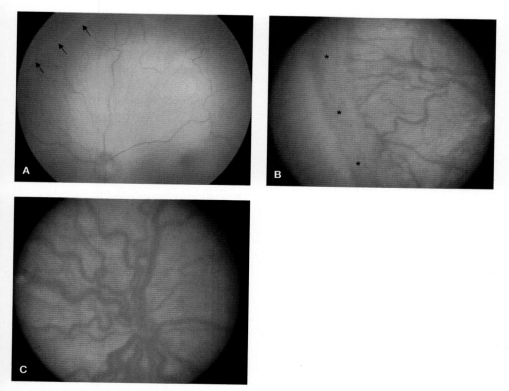

FIGURE 8-20. Retinopathy of prematurity. A. Zone II, stage 2 disease with mild to moderate plus disease. At the superior aspect of the retina, the vessel development has ceased, and a white ridge (*arrows*) is seen. Avascular, undeveloped retina is seen beyond the ridge. (Courtesy of Sharon Lehman, MD.) **B.** Zone II, stage 3 disease with plus disease. Neovascularization is seen rising into the vitreous above the ridge (*asterisks*). (Courtesy of William Tasman, MD.) **C.** Plus disease with severe vascular dilation and tortuosity. (Courtesy of William Tasman, MD.)

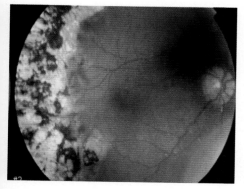

FIGURE 8-21. Retinopathy of prematurity after successful treatment with laser photocoagulation and peripheral chorioretinal scars. (Courtesy of William Tasman, MD.)

RETINITIS PIGMENTOSA

Barry N. Wasserman ■

Etiology

Retinitis pigmentosa is a group of diseases characterized by night blindness (nyctalopia), slow painless, progressive peripheral visual field loss, and progressive deterioration of the electroretinogram. Virtually every inheritance pattern has been reported and over 70 genes have been shown to be causative when mutated. Phenotypic and genetic heterogeneity are common. The common pathway is retinal receptor cell death via apoptosis. Retinitis pigmentosa may be found in isolation or in association with systemic or neurodegenerative disease.

Symptoms

Retinitis pigmentosa begins in childhood, adolescence, or early adulthood with nyctalopia and issues of light to dark adaptation. Patients may also complain of loss of peripheral vision. Other symptoms may include photophobia, variable visual acuity, and unusual colors in visual perception.

Signs

Visual acuity may range from 20/20 to no light perception but is usually preserved early in the disease. VF constriction is progressive. Posterior subcapsular cataracts are common in adult patients. Retinal findings may be minimal in children, but eventually classic "bone spicule" pattern of midperipheral hyperpigmentation occurs, with associated arteriolar thinning and waxy pallor of the optic nerve (Fig. 8-22). Other macular changes including loss of foveal reflex, irregularities of the internal limiting membrane, and cystoid maculopathy can occur. Electroretinogram findings progress to nondetectable.

Differential Diagnosis

Retinitis pigmentosa can be divided into nonsyndromic and syndromic types. Nonsyndromic types include the autosomal dominant and recessive forms, as well as X-linked forms. Rare mitochondrial DNA mutation types also occur.

Syndromic types of retinitis pigmentosa are extremely varied and include

● Syndromes associated with deafness, most commonly Usher syndrome

● Syndromes associated with metabolic diseases including Abetalipoproteinemia (Bassen-Kornzweig disease), Zellweger syndrome (cerebrohepatorenal syndrome), Refsum disease, mucopolysaccharidoses types I, II, III, and neuronal ceroid lipofuscinosis (Batten disease)

● Kearns–Sayre syndrome

● Syndromes with renal associations including Fanconi, cystinosis, Senior Loken syndrome

● Dysmorphic syndromes including Cohen syndrome, Jeune syndrome, Cockayne syndrome

● Pigmentary retinopathies: pseudo retinitis pigmentosa

● Cancer-associated retinopathy

● Congenital infections including syphilis, rubella, and CMV

● Drug-associated retinopathy including phenothiazines and chloroquine

● Retinal vascular occlusion

Diagnostic Evaluation

Ocular examination may show classic findings but may be normal early in the disease. VF testing reveals constriction, and electroretinogram shows rod and cone signals are depressed or extinguished. Contrast sensitivity is sometimes decreased. Genetic testing may be helpful for determining subtypes and prognosis.

Treatment

Genetic counseling is advised. The use of vitamin A is controversial. Oral or topical carbonic anhydrase inhibitors can be helpful for patients who have associated macular edema. Cataract extraction should be performed when indicated but may have a higher risk of postoperative cystoid macular edema. Gene therapy is under investigation. Retinal pigment epithelial transplant and electronic retinal implants are also under investigation. Low vision services are recommended as the disease progresses.

Prognosis

Visual acuity may remain better than 20/40 in over half of patients in their 40s. However, 25%

may have less than 20/200 and are considered legally blind. Only 1 in every 1000 patients come to have no light perception. X-linked types may have the worst visual acuity prognosis, whereas sector-type autosomal dominant retinitis pigmentosa patients generally retain good vision.

REFERENCES

Goodwin P. Hereditary retinal disease. *Curr Opin Ophthalmol.* 2008;19:255–262.

Grover S, Fishman GA, Anderson RJ, et al. Visual acuity impairment in patients with retinitis pigmentosa at age 45 years or older. *Ophthalmology.* 1999;106(9):1780–1785.

Hamel C. Retinitis pigmentosa. *Orphanet J Rare Dis.* 2006;1:40.

Jackson H, Garway-Heath D, Rosen P, et al. Outcome of cataract surgery in patients with retinitis pigmentosa. *Br J Ophthalmol.* 2001;85(8):936–938.

Jacobson SG, Cideciyan AV. Treatment possibilities for retinitis pigmentosa. *N Engl J Med.* 2010;363:1669–1671.

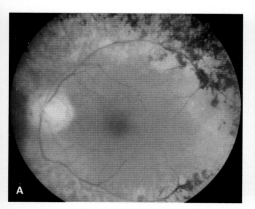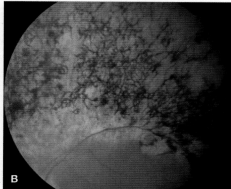

FIGURE 8-22. Retinitis pigmentosa. A. Retinitis pigmentosa fundus photos demonstrating optic nerve waxy pallor, vascular attenuation, and midperipheral "bone spicule" pigmentary retinopathy. **B.** Higher magnification photos of midperipheral "bone spicule" retinopathy.

MYELINATED NERVE FIBERS

Barry N. Wasserman ▪

Etiology

Whitish sheets or patches of myelin distributed along portions of the nerve fiber layer of the retina. Usually unilateral, myelin is produced by oligodendrocytes and is normal along the optic nerve but does not normally progress beyond the lamina cribrosa. Ectopic oligodendrocytes are associated with myelin in the retinal nerve fiber layer generally near the optic nerve. Myelinated nerve fibers may be found in 1% of eyes, and may be an isolated finding, or may be associated with other abnormalities including neurofibromatosis and Gorlin syndrome.

Symptoms

May be asymptomatic but sometimes associated with high axial myopia and amblyopia in affected eye

Signs

Poor vision on examination associated with feathery gray-white patches along the retinal nerve fiber layer. They are often found at the optic nerve and along the vascular arcades, more commonly superiorly (Fig. 8-23A). There may also be a patch unconnected to the optic nerve (Fig. 8-23B). High myopic astigmatism with anisometropic amblyopia is reported. If extensive, they can cause leukocoria (Fig. 8-24).

Differential Diagnosis

- Branch retinal artery occlusion
- Cotton wool patches
- When extensive, myelinated nerve fibers can yield leukocoria, in which case it must rule out:
  - Retinoblastoma
  - Coats disease
  - Coloboma
  - Cataract
  - ROP
  - PFV
  - FEVR

Diagnostic Evaluation

Myelinated nerve fibers are diagnosed by clinical fundus examination. Feathery gray-white patches are noted superficially in the nerve fiber layer along the vascular arcades, often in close proximity to the optic disc. VF field testing may reveal absolute or relative scotomas corresponding to the myelinated fibers. SD-OCT has shown thickening of the retinal nerve fiber layer but normal morphology of the fovea, suggesting amblyopia may be more related to anisometropia than anatomic abnormality.

Treatment

No treatment is needed for asymptomatic myelinated nerve fibers. When associated with anisometropic amblyopia, appropriate aggressive amblyopia treatment should be instituted.

Prognosis

When dense amblyopia is associated with myelinated nerve fibers, the prognosis is variable and guarded. Outcomes are worse when associated with high myopia and history of associated strabismus.

REFERENCES

Gharai S, Prakash G, Kumar DA, et al. Spectral domain optical coherence tomographic characteristics of unilateral peripapillary myelinated retinal nerve fibers involving the macula. *J AAPOS.* 2010;14:432–434.

Lee MS, Gonzalez C. Unilateral peripapillary myelinated retinal nerve fibers associated with strabismus, amblyopia, and myopia. *Am J Ophthalmol.* 1998;125:554–556.

Shelton JB, Digre KB, Gilman J, et al. Characteristics of myelinated retinal nerve fiber layer in ophthalmic imaging: findings on autofluorescence, fluorescein angiographic, infrared, optical coherence tomographic, and red-free images. *JAMA Ophthalmol.* 2013;131:107–109.

Tarabishy AB, Alexandrou TJ, Traboulsi EI. Syndrome of myelinated retinal nerve fibers, myopia, and amblyopia: a review. *Surv Ophthalmol.* 2007;52:588–596.

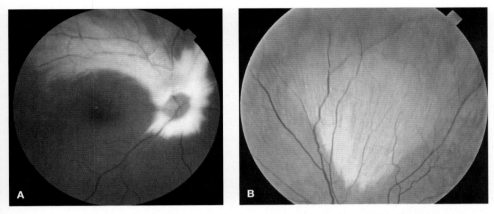

FIGURE 8-23. Myelinated nerve fibers. A. Fundus photo with extensive feathery white myelination extending in all directions from the optic nerve. **B.** Myelinated nerve fibers superior to the optic nerve without direct connection to the optic nerve. (Courtesy of William Tasman, MD.)

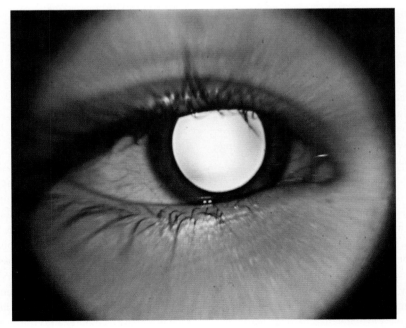

FIGURE 8-24. Myelinated nerve fibers. Leukocoria in a patient with extensive myelinated nerve fibers. (Courtesy of William Tasman, MD.)

STARGARDT DISEASE/ FUNDUS FLAVIMACULATA

Barry N. Wasserman ■

Etiology

A largely autosomal recessively inherited atrophic macular dystrophy, Stargardt disease is associated with mutations of the *ABCA4* gene on chromosome 1p. It encodes a retina-specific adenosine triphosphate-binding cassette transporter, and defects result in death of retinal pigment epithelial cells, as well as overlying photoreceptor cells. Specific mutations have not been correlated with electroretinographic characteristics or fundus appearance. This gene may also act as a modifier gene in other retinal dystrophies with other known gene mutations. Lipofuscin accumulation in the RPE is associated with vision loss. Other types of Stargardt include autosomal dominant phenotypes associated with mutations in the genes *ELOVL4* or *PROM1* and mitochondrial phenocopies.

Symptoms

Decreased central visual acuity is usually acute and precipitous in the first or second decade of life. Vision loss is sometimes seen in absence of ophthalmoscopic findings. Painless, progressive, slow visual deterioration to the 20/200 range may occur through the third decade.

Signs

Visual acuity is decreased to varying degrees at presentation. Fundus exam may be normal or only a loss of foveal reflex early in the disease, but later yellow subretinal "flecks" are seen (Fig. 8-25). Classically, the flecks are found centrally in Stargardt disease, with more profound and progressive vision loss, and in the midperiphery in fundus flavimaculata, with better

vision prognosis. Flecks have been described as "fish-scale shaped" and hence the name "pisciform." Eventually, the macula takes on a beaten bronze appearance and sometimes a bull's eye maculopathy. Fluorescein angiography may reveal a silent choroid in most patients, as the lipofuscin in the RPE blocks the appearance of dye in the choroidal vessels (Fig. 8-26). Later in the disease, there may be fluorescein hyperfluorescence in the atrophic central macula. Early electroretinogram findings may be normal, but a subset of patients do have changes with prolonged dark adaptation. Multifocal electroretinogram usually has mild abnormalities.

Differential Diagnosis

- Fundus albipunctata
- Retinitis punctata albescens
- Cone dystrophy
- Batten disease
- Hydroxychloroquine toxicity
- Autosomal dominant drusen
- Multifocal best
- Doyne honeycomb
- Sorsby dystrophy
- Malattia leventinese
- Bestrophinopathy

Diagnostic Evaluation

Decreased vision in a child, with classic dark choroid on angiography, and sometimes yellow pisciform subretinal lesions are diagnostic. VF testing most commonly reveals a central scotoma, but paracentral and other variants may be seen. Electroretinogram findings may be helpful to rule out other causes of pediatric vision loss but are often normal in early Stargardt disease. SD-OCT demonstrates hyperreflective foci not only in the retina, but also in the choroidal layers including membrane/RPE complex and choriocapillaris.

Genetic testing of the patient and other family members is often helpful.

Treatment

Genetic counseling and low vision services are recommended. No other specific treatments have proven effective to date. Avoid vitamin A supplementation.

Prognosis

Some variants of fundus flavimaculata are associated with better visual prognosis, but Stargardt disease is generally associated with moderate to poor central visual acuity.

REFERENCES

Goodwin P. Hereditary retinal disease. *Curr Opin Ophthalmol.* 2008;19:255–262.

Oh KT, Weleber RG, Stone EM, et al. Electroretinographic findings in patients with Stargardt disease and fundus flavimaculatus. *Retina.* 2004;24(6):920–928.

Piri N, Nesmith BLW, Schaal S. Choroidal hyperreflective foci in Stargardt disease shown by spectral-domain optical coherence tomography imaging: correlation with disease severity. *JAMA Ophthalmol.* 2015;133:398–405.

Testa F, Melillo P, Di Iorio V, et al. Macular function and morphologic features in juvenile Stargardt disease. *Ophthalmology.* 2014;121:2399–2405.

Westerfeld C, Mukai S. Stargardt's disease and the *ABCR* gene. *Semin Ophthalmol.* 2008;23(1):59–65.

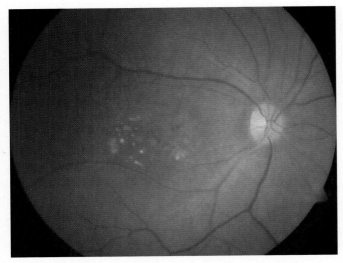

FIGURE 8-25. **Stargardt disease/fundus flavimaculata.** Fundus photos with macular yellow subretinal flecks.

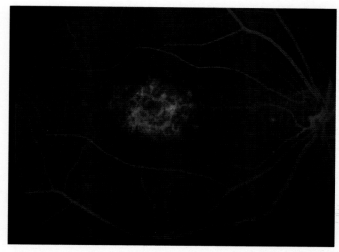

FIGURE 8-26. Stargardt disease/fundus flavimaculata. Fluorescein angiogram revealing dark or silent choroid, as lipofuscin in the retinal pigment epithelium block choroidal vessel.

Eyelid Anomalies

Kammi B. Gunton ■

ANKYLOBLEPHARON FILIFORME ADNATUM

Etiology

- Ectodermal dysplasia, temporary epithelial arrest, and rapid mesenchymal proliferation allow fusion of eyelid margin. Normal eyelids are only fused until the fifth gestational month.

- May be sporadic or associated with three ectodermal syndromes: ankyloblepharon-ectodermal dysplasia-clefting (AEC) (*TP63* gene deficits), popliteal pterygium syndrome with webbing in lower limbs (*IRF6* gene deficits), or curly hair-ankyloblepharon-nail dysplasia

- Has also been associated with meningocele, hydrocephalus, patent ductus arteriosis or ventral septal defects, iridogoniodysgenesis with glaucoma, imperforate anus, bilateral syndactyly

Symptoms

- Inability to open eye
- May occur unilaterally or bilaterally

Signs

- Partial or complete fusion of eyelid margins along portion of their length by webs of skin (**Fig. 9-1**) arise from gray line anterior to the meibomian glands and posterior to the cilia

- Shortened vertical palpebral fissure

Differential Diagnosis

- Cryptophthalmos, failure of differentiation of eyelid structures; the cornea is attached to eyelid skin

- Congenital coloboma, defect within the eyelid, small notch or entire eyelid absent

- Epiblepharon, with extra fold of orbicularis, in the lower eyelid, turning eyelashes inward; no attachment between eyelids

Diagnostic Evaluation

- External examination of the eyelids reveals strands or a web of skin attaching the eyelid margin.

- Underlying cornea and eye structures are intact and unaffected.

- Consultation for associated ectodermal and other conditions

- Molecular genetic testing for *TP63* or *IRF6* mutations if indicated

Treatment

- Spontaneous resolution may occur, but surgical incision may be needed to prevent amblyopia.

- Hemostat to connective tissue followed by excision of skin strands or webs. Edges of conjunctiva and eyelid margin are apposed with sutures to prevent readhesion of skin.

Prognosis

- Excellent prognosis with treatment

REFERENCES

Alami B, Maadane A, Sekhsoukh R. Ankyloblepharon filiforme adnatum: a case report. *Pan Afr Med J.* 2013;15:15.

Jain S, Atkinson A, Hopkisson B. Ankyloblepharon filiforme adnatum. *Br J Ophthalmol.* 1997;81(8):705.

Lopardo T, Loiacono N, Marinari B, et al. Claudin-1 is a p63 target gene with a crucial role in epithelial development. *PLoS One.* 2008;3(7):e2715.

Scott MH, Richard JM, Farris BK. Ankyloblepharon filiforme adnatum associated with infantile glaucoma and iridogoniodysgenesis. *J Pediatr Ophthalmol Strabismus.* 1994;31(2):93–95.

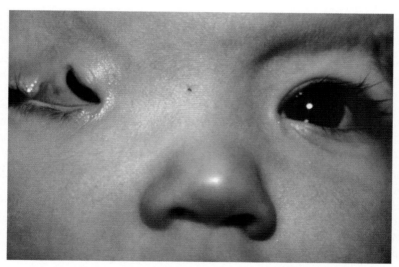

FIGURE 9-1. Ankyloblepharon with coloboma, right eyelid. (Courtesy of Robert Penne, MD, Department of Oculoplastics, Wills Eye Hospital, Philadelphia.)

BLEPHAROPHIMOSIS, PTOSIS, AND EPICANTHUS INVERSUS SYNDROME (BPES)

Etiology

- Autosomal dominant inheritance
- Associated with *FOXL2* mutations, commonly autosomal dominant

Symptoms

- Present congenitally
- Severe ptosis may cause ametropic amblyopia with blurred vision
- Chin-up head posture

Signs

- Shortened horizontal palpebral fissure with three associated major signs: telecanthus (widened intercanthal distance with normal interpupillary distance), epicanthus inversus (skin fold from lower eyelid running upward), and severe ptosis (Fig. 9-2)
- Additional signs include lower eyelid entropion, a poorly developed nasal bridge, hypoplasia of superior orbital rim, low-set ears, a short philtrum, refractive errors, strabismus, amblyopia, hypertelorism, laterally displaced inferior punctum in lower eyelid, abnormal intelligence with larger genetic rearrangements in *FOXL2* gene.
- Type I BPES (blepharophimosis, ptosis, epicanthus inversus syndrome) is associated with ovarian dysfunction, leading to premature ovarian failure.
- Type II BPES—classic features with no other associations

Differential Diagnosis

- Congenital ptosis: would occur with absence of other features
- Epicanthus, isolated finding

Diagnostic Evaluation

- Based on the presence of four classic signs: blepharophimosis, ptosis, epicanthus inversus, and telecanthus
- Ophthalmic evaluation for associated conditions
- Genetic testing for *FOXL2* to assess risk of ovarian dysfunction
- Referral to endocrinologist for ovarian dysfunction if indicated, pelvic ultrasound, bone density assessment

Treatment

- Staged surgical treatment of signs, medial canthoplasty including double Z or Y-V-plasty and intranasal wiring of medial canthus tendons to correct telecanthus at age 3 to 5 followed later by bilateral frontalis sling or levator resection as indicated for ptosis. With bilateral ametropic amblyopia, ptosis repair may need to be expedited.
- Simultaneous medial canthoplasty and blepharoptosis correction in select patients and correction of lower eyelid transposition may be helpful.

Prognosis

- With surgical correction, improved cosmesis is achieved.
- Visual prognosis is guarded because of amblyopia development. Timing of surgical correction is critical to prevent amblyopia.

- Ovarian dysfunction is treated with hormone replacement therapy, and reproductive issues may be addressed with reproductive technologies, including embryo or egg donation.

REFERENCES

Decock CE, Claerhout I, Leroy BP, Kesteleyn P, Shah AD, De Baere E. Correction of the lower eyelid malpositioning in the blepharophimosis-ptosis-epicanthus inversus syndrome. *Ophthal Plast Reconstr Surg.* 2011;27:368–370.

Sebastiá R, Herzog Neto G, Fallico E, Lessa S, Solari HP, Ventura MP. A one-stage correction of the blepharophimosis syndrome using a standard combination of surgical techniques. *Aesthetic Plast Surg.* 2011;35:820–827.

Verdin H, DeBaere E. Blepharophimosis, ptosis and epicanthus inversus. In: Pagon RA, Adam MP, Ardinger HH, et al, eds. *GeneReviews.* Seattle: University of Washington; 2015.

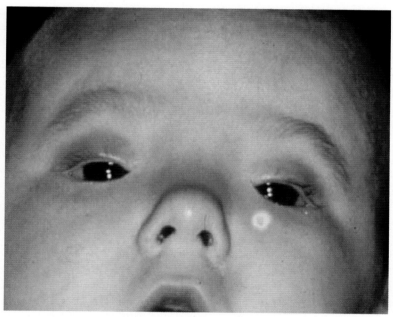

FIGURE 9-2. Child with blepharophimosis syndrome. Note blepharophimosis with telecanthus (widened intercanthal distance), epicanthus inversus, and severe ptosis. (Courtesy of Robert Penne, MD, Department of Oculoplastics, Wills Eye Hospital, Philadelphia.)

CHILDHOOD ECTROPION

Etiology

- Congenital or acquired
- Congenital resulting from absence or atrophy of tarsal plate and anterior lamella
- Acquired resulting from paralytic, cicatricial, or mechanical causes in childhood with vertical shortening of anterior lamella such as congenital malformations with skin retraction, floppy eyelid syndrome, trauma, burns, ichthyosis (cicatricial), inflammatory conditions from medications, bilateral eyelid eversion during delivery, allergies with orbicularis spasm, or tumors (mechanical)
- May occur in association with BPES, euryblepharon, microphthalmos, orbital cysts, and Down syndrome

Symptoms

- Chronic epiphora, conjunctival injection/ chemosis, foreign body sensation, photophobia, reduced vision

Signs

- Eversion of eyelid margin; lower eyelid is more commonly involved because of a vertical deficiency of skin (**Fig. 9-3**)
- Exposure keratitis and conjunctivitis

Differential Diagnosis

- Congenital tarsal kink: upper eyelid bent back with 180-degree fold of the upper tarsal plate
- Congenital entropion: distal portion of lower tarsal plate bent inward

- Euryblepharon: downward displacement of temporal portion of lower eyelid caused by enlargement of the lateral aperture

Diagnostic Evaluation

- Based on external examination with eversion of the eyelid

Treatment

- Mild cases require lubrication with artificial tears or ointments.
- With corneal exposure, surgical repair is required with lateral tarsorrhaphy or lateral canthoplasty to eliminate horizontal eyelid laxity to reposition the eyelid to the globe.
- In severe cases, a full-thickness skin graft is required.
- In tarsus agenesis, a uricular cartilage may be used in the graft.

Prognosis

- With surgical correction, and skin graft in cases of vertical deficiency of skin, there is good prognosis.
- Must prevent permanent corneal scarring from exposure keratitis, with resulting amblyopia

REFERENCES

Bedran EG, Pereira MV, Bernandes TF. Ectropion. *Semin Ophthalmol.* 2010;25:59–65.

Cavuoto KM, Hui JI. Congenital eyelid eversion. *J Pediatr Ophthalmol Strabismus.* 2010;47:Online:e1-3 doi:10.3928/01913913-20100507-02.

Fea A, Turco D, Actis AG, et al. Ectropion, entropion, trichasis. *Minerva Chir.* 2013;68:27–35.

Piskiniene R. Eyelid malposition: lower lid entropion and ectropion. *Medicina (Kaunas).* 2006;42:881–884.

Vallabhanath P, Carter S. Ectropion and entropion. *Curr Opinion Ophthalmol.* 2000;11:345–351.

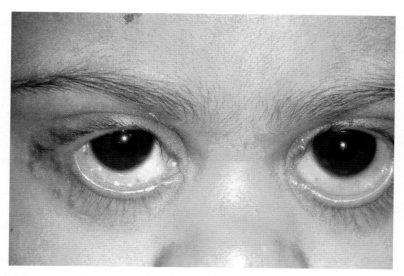

FIGURE 9-3. Ectropion. Note eversion of lower eyelids. (Courtesy of Jacqueline Carrasco, MD, Department of Oculoplastics, Wills Eye Hospital, Philadelphia.)

CONGENITAL ENTROPION

Etiology

- Congenital or acquired
- Congenital from retractor dysgenesis and shortened posterior lamella, absence or kinking in tarsal plate
- Acquired from acute spastic, involutional and cicatricial from trachoma, Stevens-Johnson syndrome, herpes zoster, chemical injury, toxic reaction to topical medications
- Involutional entropion is more common in Asians
- Often associated with epiblepharon, epicanthus, microphthalmos, and enophthalmos

Symptoms

- Epiphora, eyelid rubbing, photophobia
- Foreign body sensation, eye pain, conjunctival injection, reduced vision

Signs

- Inward turning of eyelid
- Lower eyelid more commonly affected
- No skin fold in eyelid (**Fig. 9-4**)
- Corneal abrasion or keratitis from eyelash abrasions

Differential Diagnosis

- Trichiasis
- Epicanthus
- Epiblepharon

Diagnostic Evaluation

- External examination reveals inward turning of the eyelid margin.
- Evaluation for presence of the tarsal plate or etiology of entropion

Treatment

- Lubrication to prevent keratitis until surgical correction
- Excision of horizontal strip of orbicularis 3 mm from the eyelid border with suturing of lower eyelid retractors to tarsus stops the preseptal orbicularis from riding over the pretarsal portion.
- Upper eyelid entropion treated with excision of skin and orbicularis to tarsus and rotation of lid margin (Weis procedure)
- Other surgical procedures include everting (Quickert) sutures and orbicularis transfer technique.

Prognosis

- Prevention of corneal scarring yields a good prognosis.
- Risk for amblyopia and refractive error

REFERENCES

Katowitz WR, Katowitz JA. Congenital and developmental eyelid abnormalities. *Plast Reconstr Surg.* 2009; 124(suppl):93e–105e.

Pereira MG, Rodrigues MA, Rodrigues SA. Eyelid entropion. *Semin Ophthalmol.* 2010;25:52–58.

Takahashi Y, Ikeda H, Ichinose A, Kakizaki H. Congenital entropion: outcome of posterior layer advancement of lower eyelid retractors and histological study of orbicularis oculi muscle hypertrophy. *Orbit.* 2014;33:444–448.

Vahdani K, Konstandinidis A, Thaller VT. A simple new technique for treatment of tarsal kink syndrome. *Ophthal Plast Reconstr Surg.* 2017;33(3S suppl 1):S77–S79.

Vallabhanath P, Carter S. Ectropion and entropion. *Curr Opinion Ophthalmol.* 2000;11:345–351.

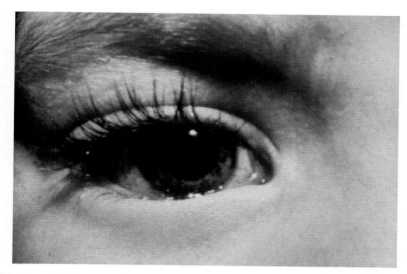

FIGURE 9-4. **Congenital entropion.** Inversion of the lower eyelid. (From Levin AV, Wilson TW, Pashby R, et al. Lids and adnexa. In: Levin AV, Wilson T, eds. *The Hospital for Sick Children's Atlas of Pediatric Ophthalmology.* Philadelphia, PA: Lippincott Williams & Wilkins; 2007:31–39.)

CONGENITAL PTOSIS

Etiology

● Unilateral and most commonly isolated finding, 35% associated with genetic, chromosomal, or neurologic conditions

● Most histologic studies support dysgenesis of levator palpebrae superioris muscle or innervational abnormalities.

● Equal frequency among different races and between sexes

Symptoms

● Asymmetry of eyelid position

● Amblyopia 1% to 12% prevalence in ptosis

Signs

● Vertical shortening of the palpebral fissure caused by upper eyelid droop (Fig. 9-5)

● Normal upper eyelid position is 1 to 2 mm below the superior limbus.

● Chin-up posture for distance viewing

Differential Diagnosis

● Marcus-Gunn jaw wink, anomalous eyelid synkineses

● Chronic progressive external ophthalmoplegia

● Third nerve palsy

● Horner syndrome

● Congenital fibrosis of extraocular muscles, congenital cranial dysinnervation disorder

● Myasthenia gravis

Diagnostic Evaluation

● Evaluation of eyelid position, margin–corneal reflex distance, levator excursion, presence of eyelid crease, notation of any abnormal head posture

● Refractive error, amblyopia assessment

● Evaluate for extraocular muscle functions, especially superior rectus and synergistic eye movements as well as pupillary response and symmetry

Treatment

● Multiple surgical treatments available depending on the degree of levator function and amount of droop, including frontalis sling; levator resection; Whitnall sling; and in limited cases with mild ptosis, Müllerectomy

Prognosis

● Evaluation for anisometropic amblyopia

● Refractive error does not significantly change following ptosis surgery.

● Concern for corneal exposure into adulthood, especially in the absence of Bell phenomenon

● Recurrence of ptosis with facial growth, laxity in sutures for frontal sling

REFERENCES

Byard SD, Sood V, Jones CA. Long-term refractive changes in children following ptosis surgery: a case series and a review of the literature. *Int Ophthalmol.* 2014;34:1303–1307.

Finsterer J. Ptosis: causes, presentation, and management. *Aesthetic Plast Surg.* 2003;27:193–204.

Ho YF, Wu SY, Tsai YJ. Factors associated with surgical outcomes in congenital ptosis: a 10-year study of 319 cases. *Am J Ophthalmol.* 2017;175:173–182.

Stein A, Kelly JP, Weiss AH. Congenital eyelid ptosis: onset and prevalence of amblyopia, associations with systemic disorders and treatment outcomes. *J Pediatr.* 2014;165:820–824.

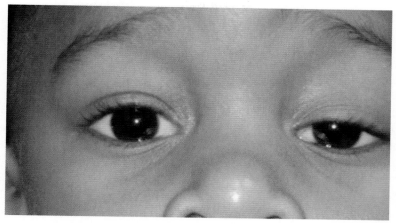

FIGURE 9-5. **Congenital ptosis.** Congenital ptosis of the left eye.

EYELID COLOBOMAS

Etiology

- Localized failure of fusion of embryonic eyelid folds, failure of adhesion of eyelid folds, or dehiscence of fused eyelid due to inadequate migration of mesenchyme into ectodermal fold, trauma from amniotic bands

- More common for upper eyelid to be affected and occurs unilaterally, one-third isolated, remainder associated with ocular or craniofacial abnormality

- Associated syndromes include CHARGE, Fraser syndrome, Goldenhar syndrome (oculo-auriculo-vertebral spectrum), craniofacial dysostosis, clefting disorders, amniotic band sequence, neurocutaneous syndromes, iris and fundus coloboma

- No inheritance pattern for isolated upper eyelid coloboma; loose dominant hereditary pattern for lower eyelid coloboma; syndromes with genetic associations

Symptoms

- Epiphora with corneal, conjunctival exposure especially in upper eyelid coloboma

Signs

- Defect in eyelid margin; varies from small defect to absence of length of eyelid (Fig. 9-6)

- Isolated upper eyelid defect may be quadrangular or triangular and at junction of medial and central parts of the eyelid

- Edges of defect rounded and covered with conjunctiva

- Corneal epithelial erosion and ulceration with large coloboma

Differential Diagnosis

- Euryblepharon
- Congenital ectropion
- Tarsal kink

Diagnostic Evaluation

- External examination with complete absence of portion of eyelid margin, including eyelashes

- Assessment for associated ocular abnormalities, symblepharon, choristomas, iris or fundus coloboma, microphthalmia

- Consultation for associated syndrome and genetic workup if applicable

Treatment

- Up to one-third eyelid margin repaired with direct closure; lateral cantholysis can provide horizontal relaxation required for closure

- Eyelid sharing procedures such as Cutler-Beard and Hughes in children occlude visual axis, albeit temporarily, and may result in amblyopia

Prognosis

- Cosmesis guarded depending on size of defect

- Prevent corneal scarring to prevent amblyopia

REFERENCES

Smith HB, Verity DH, O'Collin JR. The incidence, embryology, and oculofacial abnormalities associated with eyelid colobomas. *Eye*. 2015;29:492–498.

Tawfik HA, Abdulhafez MH, Fouad YA. Congenital upper eyelid coloboma: embryologic, nomenclatorial, nosologic, etiologic, pathogenetic, epidemiologic, clinical and management perspectives. *Ophthal Plast Reconstr Surg*. 2015;31:1–12.

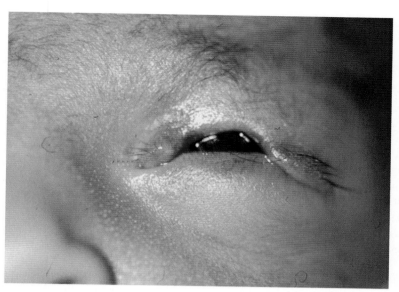

FIGURE 9-6. Upper eyelid coloboma. (Courtesy of Robert Penne, MD, Department of Oculoplastics, Wills Eye Hospital, Philadelphia.)

EPIBLEPHARON

Etiology

- Overriding pretarsal orbicularis with horizontal skin layer pushing the cilia vertically

- Possible etiologies for redundant skin include a weak attachment of the pretarsal orbicularis to the tarsus, hypertrophy of the orbicularis oculi, or failure of septae in the subcutaneous plane of the pretarsal orbicularis and overlying skin, resulting in poor adhesion between the lower eyelid retractors and skin or orbicularis.

- More common in Asians, involving lower eyelid, and bilateral

Symptoms

- Possibly none or vertical orientation of eyelashes

- Severe cases: foreign body sensation, epiphora, conjunctival injection, photophobia, eyelid rubbing

Signs

- Presence of excess horizontal skin along the upper or lower eyelid margin that forces cilia into a vertical position, often against ocular surface with blink (**Fig. 9-7**)

- Tarsus in a normal position relative to the globe

- Corneal epithelial defects in severe cases

Differential Diagnosis

- Entropion: eyelid turned inward relative to the globe

Diagnostic Evaluation

- External examination with eyelid margin in normal position relative to the globe; excess horizontal skin fold pushing cilia toward the globe into a vertical position

- Evaluation of the cornea for staining

Treatment

- In the absence of corneal pathology, no treatment is indicated. Subsequently, facial growth frequently eliminates condition.

- Appropriate lubrication with ointments to protect corneal surface before surgical correction when corneal keratitis is detected.

- If required, horizontal skin from the eyelid margin is excised with the underlying orbicularis; reapproximation of the skin edges, pulling the cilia away from the ocular surface, is made.

- Alternatively, the above procedure is combined with thermal cautery to the orbital septum or a rotating suture allowing adhesion of the septum to the preseptal orbicularis and preventing overriding of muscle and sutures in the inferior tarsus and upper skin flap to further rotate cilia from ocular surface

Prognosis

- Spontaneous resolution in the majority of cases with facial growth (90%)

- Primary excision of pretarsal orbicularis is highly effective; patients with Down syndrome may have a slightly higher recurrence rate.

REFERENCES

Kakizaki H, Leibovitch I, Takahashi Y, et al. Eyelash inversion in epiblepharon: is it caused by redundant skin? *Clin Ophthalmol.* 2009;3:247–250.

Kim JS, Jin SW, Hur MC, et al. The clinical characteristics and surgical outcomes of epiblepharon in Korean children: a 9-year experience. *J Ophthalmol.* 2014;2014:156501.

Lee KM, Choung HK, Kim NJ, et al. Prognosis of upper eyelid epiblepharon repair in Down syndrome. *Am J Ophthalmol.* 2010;150:476–480.e1.

Woo KI, Kim YD. Management of epiblepharon: state of the art. *Curr Opin Ophthalmol.* 2016;27:433–438.

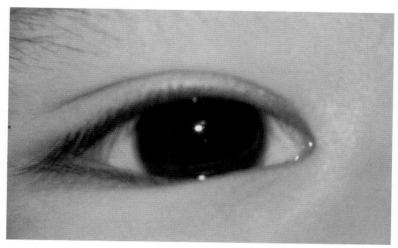

FIGURE 9-7. Epiblepharon. Note the excess horizontal skin in the lower eyelid margin pushing cilia into a vertical position. (Courtesy of Alex Levin, MD, Department of Pediatric Ophthalmology, Wills Eye Hospital, Philadelphia.)

EPICANTHUS

Etiology

- Usually bilateral; can be isolated or associated with ptosis or BPES, especially epicanthus inversus

- More common in Asians

- Histologic studies show possible congenital dysplasia of the medial canthal tendon with disorganized collagen in BPES contributing to epicanthus.

Symptoms

- None

Signs

- Semilunar fold of skin extending from upper eyelid medially to the margin of the lower eyelid

- Four types:

  - Tarsalis: fold of skin most prominent in upper eyelid; most common (Fig. 9-8)

  - Inversus: skin fold arises from below the canthus; prominent in lower eyelid

  - Palpebralis: fold equally distributed between the upper and lower eyelids

  - Supraciliaris: skin fold originates above the canthus from the eyebrow region

Differential Diagnosis

- BPES

- Hypertelorism; enlarged bony distance between orbits

Diagnostic Evaluation

- External examination of eyelids with notation of skin fold origination site and prominent eyelid involvement

Treatment

- Most often none required; facial growth diminishes appearance, unless epicanthus inversus

- If desired, after facial maturity, reconstruction of eyelid is recommended; in epicanthus palpebralis and inversus a Y-V procedure, in epicanthus tarsalis, a small V-Y procedure at inner canthus; in severe epicanthus inversus a double Z may be indicated.

Prognosis

- Good cosmesis with surgical correction if required

REFERENCES

Johnson CC. Developmental abnormalities of the eyelids. *Ophthalmic Plast Reconstr Surg.* 1986;2:219–232.

Katowitz WR, Katowitz JA. Congenital and developmental eyelid abnormalities. *Plast Reconstr Surg.* 2009;124(suppl):93e–105e.

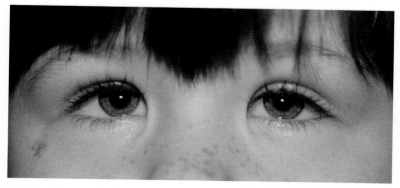

FIGURE 9-8. **Epicanthus tarsalis.** (Courtesy of Alex Levin, MD, Department of Pediatric Ophthalmology, Wills Eye Hospital, Philadelphia.)

CAPILLARY HEMANGIOMAS

Etiology

- Most common vascular orbital benign tumor of childhood
- Unencapsulated lesion with lobules of endothelial cells lining blood-filled spaces with intervening fibrous septa
- More common in females
- Present at birth to several months of life; rapid growth for 3 to 6 months in the proliferative phase followed by quiescence for few years, and then involutional phase with fibrofatty deposition around endothelial cells with fibrosis and involution of the lesion
- During the proliferative phase, basic fibroblast growth factor (bFGF) and vascular endothelial growth factor (VEGF) play a role.

Symptoms

- Blurred vision, ptosis, skin lesion

Signs

- Classic superficial strawberry nevus mass lesion in the skin (Fig. 9-9)
- Subcutaneous, blue- to purple-colored mass lesion in the orbit
- Proptosis without skin discoloration from deep orbital hemangiomas
- Reduced vision; anisometropic astigmatism

Differential Diagnosis

- Lymphangioma: no overlying strawberry nevus, episodic hemorrhages around orbit
- Rhabdomyosarcoma: rapid growth with proptosis
- Orbital dermoid: classic superotemporal location, slow growth

Diagnostic Evaluation

- External examination and imaging study as needed to determine the extent of the hemangioma
- Systemic evaluation for Kasabach-Merritt syndrome with thrombocytopenia and Posterior fossa brain malformations, Hemangioma, Arterial lesions (head or neck), Cardia abnormalities, and Eye abnormalities (glaucoma, microphthalmia, optic nerve hypoplasia, among others) (PHACE) syndrome

Treatment

- In the presence of amblyopia, options for treatment include oral steroids, intralesional steroids, argon laser, injection of sclerosing agents, surgical excision, and oral and perhaps topical propranolol
- Propranolol 2 mg/kg/day divided three times a day; response in size at 24 hours. Extend oral treatment for 12 months. Propranolol causes rapid vasoconstriction and may reduce expression of VEGF and bFGF or promote apoptosis of capillary endothelial cells to reduce the hemangioma. Possible side effects of propranolol include bradycardia, hypotension, and hypoglycemia, so monitoring is required. Residual scarring may occur with treatment.
- Topical 0.25% timolol gel twice daily showed good response in 60% of cases; not effective in deep orbital lesions

Prognosis

- The involutional phase occurs over 5 to 7 years. Complete resolution occurs in 75% to 90% of children by age 7.
- Amblyopia is difficult to treat and more common in upper eyelid lesions, nasal eyelid location, lesions larger than 1 cm, and diffuse orbital lesions.

REFERENCES

Chambers CB, Katowitz WR, Katowitz JA, Binenbaum G. A controlled study of topical 0.25% timolol maleate gel for the treatment of cutaneous infantile capillary hemangiomas. *Ophthalmic Plast Reconstru Surg.* 2012;28:103–106.

Hernandez JA, Chia A, Quah BL, Seah LL. Periocular capillary hemangioma: management practices in recent years. *Clin Ophthalmol.* 2013;7:1227–1232.

Leaute-Labreze C, Dumas de la Roque E, Hubiche T, et al. Propranolol for severe hemangiomas of infancy. *N Engl J Med.* 2008;358:2649–2651.

Schwartz SR, Blei F, Ceisler E, et al. Risk factors for amblyopia in children with capillary hemangiomas of the eyelids and orbit. *J AAPOS.* 2006;10:262–268.

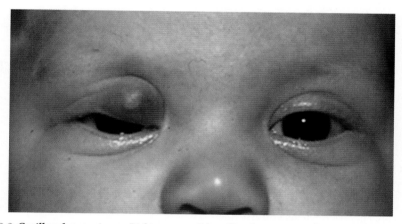

FIGURE 9-9. Capillary hemangioma. Right upper eyelid capillary hemangioma. (Courtesy of Judith Lavrich, MD, Department of Pediatric Ophthalmology, Wills Eye Hospital, Philadelphia.)

CHAPTER 10

Lacrimal Anomalies

Bruce M. Schnall, Leonard B. Nelson, and Emily Schnall ■

CONGENITAL NASOLACRIMAL DUCT OBSTRUCTION

- Congenital nasolacrimal duct obstruction (NLDO) is the most common abnormality of infants' lacrimal apparatus, occurring in 6% of infants.

Etiology

- Sporadic
- An imperforate membrane at the distal level of the nasolacrimal duct is the usual cause of occlusion.

Symptoms

- Usually presents within the first weeks of life with epiphora and crusting on lashes
- Discharge in an eye without conjunctival injection

Signs

- Typically, the tears spill over the lower eyelid, and there is a "wet look" in the involved eye(s) (Fig. 10-1).
- Eyelashes may be matted together from mucus discharge.

- Conjunctiva usually appears white and uninflamed.

Diagnostic Evaluation

- Clinical history, symptoms, and signs are usually enough to establish diagnosis.
- Can perform fluorescein dye disappearance test (Fig. 10-2)
- May be mimicked by other disorders that cause excessive tearing such as infantile glaucoma

Treatment

- Although controversy continues to exist, most studies have shown spontaneous remittance in 80% to 90% of affected infants by 12 months of age.
- Massage, eyelid hygiene, and occasional antibiotic treatment
- If symptoms are still present by 13 months of age, probing is recommended (Fig. 10-3).
- If repeated probing is necessary and does not eliminate symptoms, the patient may require intubation with silicone tubing or balloon catheter.

Prognosis

- Most congenital NLDOs resolve spontaneously before age 1 and do not need probing.

- Most NLDOs that require probing are cured with that procedure and do not require an intubation or balloon catheter.

REFERENCES

El-Mansoury J, Calhoun JH, Nelson LB, et al. Results of late probing for congenital nasolacrimal duct obstruction. *Ophthalmology.* 1986;93:1052–1054.

Nelson LB, Calhoun JH, Menduke H. Medical management of congenital nasolacrimal duct obstruction. *J Pediatric Ophthalmol Strabismus.* 1985;76:172–175.

Pediatric Eye Disease Investigator Group. Primary treatment of nasolacrimal duct obstruction with nasolacrimal duct intubation in children less than four years old. *J AAPOS.* 2008;12:445–450.

Pediatric Eye Disease Investigator Group. Balloon catheter dilation and nasolacrimal duct intubation for treatment of nasolacrimal duct obstruction after failed probing. *Arch Ophthalmol.* 2009;127(5):633–639.

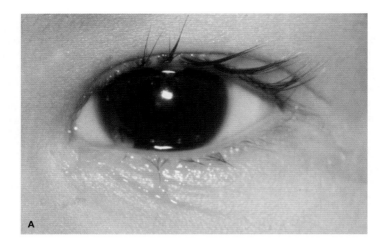

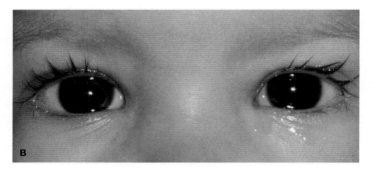

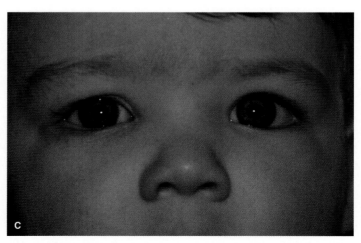

FIGURE 10-1. **Nasolacrimal duct obstruction.** **A.** Nasolacrimal duct obstruction (NLDO) showing the "wet look," with matting of the lashes. **B.** Bilateral NLDO, tearing, and matting of the lashes. Notice that the conjunctiva is clear. **C.** Right NLDO, no obstruction on left. Notice lashes are matted on right eye only.

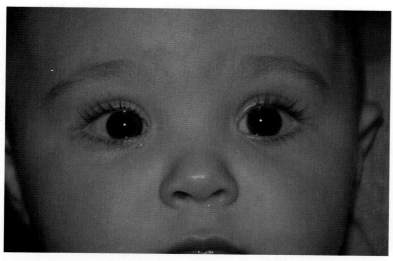

FIGURE 10-2. Nasolacrimal duct obstruction. Dye disappearance test with photograph taken 10 minutes after placing fluorescein dye in both eyes. Fluorescein remains in right eye indicating right nasolacrimal duct is obstructed. Fluorescein has drained from left eye into the nose and can be seen draining from the left nares indicating the left nasolacrimal duct is patent.

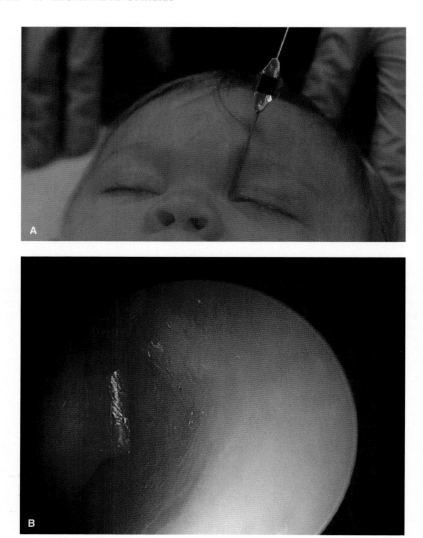

FIGURE 10-3. Nasolacrimal system probing. A. Probe in the lacrimal system. **B.** Probe buried under nasal mucosa of the inferior turbinate at time of probing viewed by nasal endoscopy. Frequently, a "pop" can be felt as the probe breaks through the nasal mucosa.

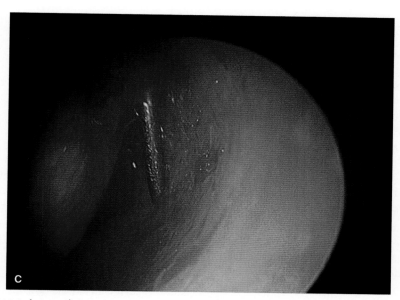

FIGURE 10-3. (*continued*) **C.** Probe has now broken through the nasal mucosa and can be see exiting under the inferior turbinate.

DACRYOCELE

- An obstruction proximally and distally in the lacrimal system of a newborn causing the lacrimal sac to swell, appearing as a mass in the lower lid nasally. The valve of Hasner distends into the nose, producing an intranasal cyst. It is also referred to as amniotocele and congenital mucocele.

Etiology

- Sporadic
- Membrane at the valve of Hasner (where the lacrimal system enters the nose) and ball valve effect at the valve of Rosenmüller (entrance of canaliculi into the lacrimal sac) allow fluid to accumulate in the lacrimal system causing the lacrimal sac to enlarge. This accumulating fluid distends the membrane at the valve of Hasner into the nose, producing an intranasal cyst.
- Usually present at birth—however, may begin in the first few weeks of life.

Symptoms

- Tearing
- Difficulty breathing from associated intranasal cyst
- Difficulty with breastfeeding on the mother's breast ipsilateral to the mucocele

Signs

- Blue-gray swelling inferior to the medial canthal tendon at birth (Fig. 10-4)
- Distended lacrimal sac will displace the medial canthal tendon superiorly, causing the lid fissure to slant upward nasally.
- Secondary infection (erythema of the tissues overlying the lacrimal sac) may occur (Fig. 10-5).
- Will extend intranasally as a submucocele mass beneath the inferior turbinate (Fig. 10-6)

Differential Diagnosis

- Hemangioma
- Dermoid
- Encephalocele
- Nasal glioma
- Phakomatous choristoma

Treatment

- Oftentimes will resolve within a few days with massage, warm compresses, and topical antibiotics
- Dacryocystitis can develop rapidly and requires IV antibiotics and hospitalization.
- If the dacryocele cannot be decompressed with massage, within several days, prompt probing with excision of the associated intranasal cyst with nasal endoscopy is recommended. Rarely, serious complications of central nervous system infections have been reported; therefore, some have recommended early probing.
- Infected dacryoceles should be treated with 24 hours of IV antibiotics before probing and excision of intranasal cyst.

Prognosis

- The resolution rate with conservative management is approximately 76%.
- Probing with intranasal cyst excision has been reported to have a 95% success rate.

REFERENCES

Harris GJ, DiClementi D. Congenital dacryocystocele. *Arch Ophthalmol.* 1982;100:1763–1765.

Paysee EA, Coats DK, Bernstein JM, et al. Management and complications of congenital dacryocele with concurrent intranasal mucocele. *J AAPOS.* 2000;4:46–53.

Schnall BM, Christian CJ. Conservative treatment of congenial dacryocele. *J Pediatr Ophthalmol Strabismus.* 1996;33:219–222.

Shekunov J, Griepentrog GJ, Diehl NN, Mohney BG. Prevalence and clinical characteristics of congenital dacryocystocele. *J AAPOS.* 2010;14:417–420.

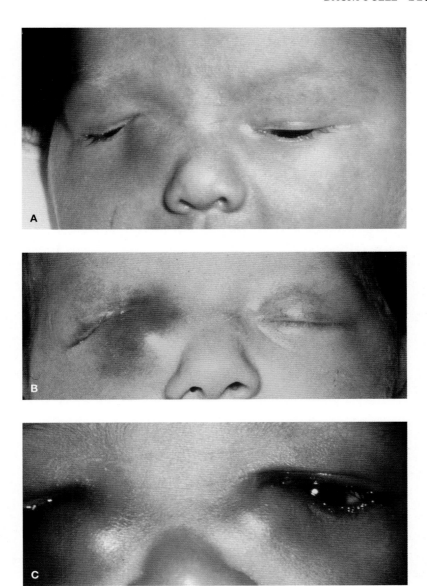

FIGURE 10-4. Dacryocele. A. Dacryocele of the nasolacrimal system showing swelling and mild erythema. The lid fissure slants upward nasally. **B.** Dacryocele showing more significant swelling and erythema. **C.** Bilateral dacryoceles.

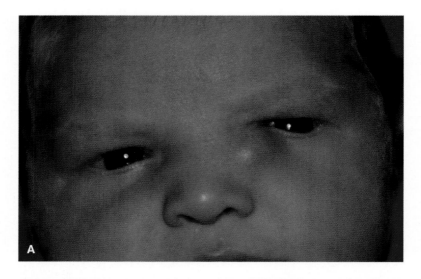

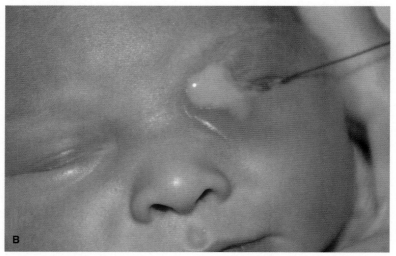

FIGURE 10-5. Dacryocele. A. Congenital dacryocele before probing. **B.** Same patient at time of office probing with a large amount of material draining from the lacrimal sac.

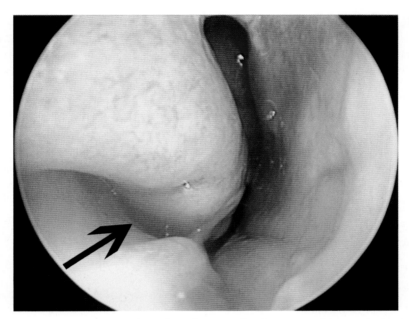

FIGURE 10-6. Dacryocele. Intranasal cyst (*arrow*) associated with a congenital dacryocele viewed by nasal endoscopy at the time of probing. This intranasal cyst is excised at the time of probing.

LACRIMAL FISTULA

- An epithelial-lined tract from the lacrimal system to the overlying skin

Etiology

- Congenital

- Likely occurs during embryogenesis with the canalization of a cord of epithelial cells from the lacrimal sac or common canaliculus to the skin

Symptoms

- Usually asymptomatic but may be associated with tearing or discharge

Signs

- Appears as an umbilication in the skin inferonasal to the medial canthus (Fig. 10-7)

Diagnostic Evaluation

- Clinical appearance is usually enough to establish diagnosis. Probing the fistula can demonstrate its connection to the lacrimal system.

Treatment

- If asymptomatic, no treatment is needed.

- If associated with discharge or tearing, the fistula tract can be closed with cautery or excised and the lacrimal system probed.

Prognosis

- Most congenital lacrimal fistula do not require treatment.

REFERENCE

Birchansky LD, Nerad JA, Kersten RC, et al. Management of congenital lacrimal sac fistula. *Arch Ophthalmol.* 1990;108:388–390.

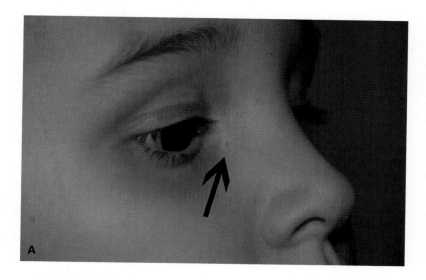

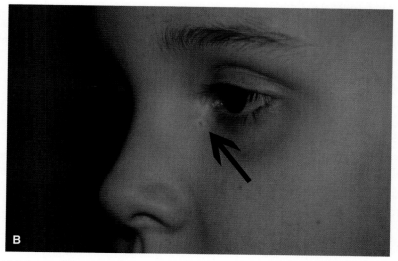

FIGURE 10-7. Lacrimal fistula. **A.** Congenital lacrimal fistula (*arrow*) appearing as an umbilication inferonasal to medial canthus. **B.** Same patient with congenital lacrimal fistula (*arrow*) in the left eye.

CHAPTER

11

Strabismus Disorders

Scott E. Olitsky and Leonard B. Nelson ∎

PSEUDOESOTROPIA

Epidemiology and Etiology

● Pseudoesotropia is one of the most common reasons an ophthalmologist is asked to evaluate an infant. In some series, up to half of children with suspected strabismus were found to have pseudoesotropia.

● Pseudoesotropia is characterized by the false appearance of strabismus when the visual axes are actually aligned (Fig. 11-1).

History

● Pseudoesotropia is usually caused by a flat, broad nasal bridge; prominent epicanthal folds; or a narrow interpupillary distance. An observer may perceive less white sclera nasally than would be expected, and the impression is that the eye is turned in toward the nose, especially when the child looks to either side.

Differential Diagnosis

● Small-angle strabismus
● Intermittent strabismus

Diagnostic Evaluation

● Pseudoesotropia can be differentiated from true strabismus when the corneal light reflex is seen to be centered in both eyes or when the cover–uncover test shows no refixation movement.

● Tightening the epicanthal folds by pinching the bridge of the nose can also be effective in demonstrating that the "crossing" is not real.

● A complete evaluation should be performed, including cycloplegic refraction, to rule out excessive hyperopia that could be causing intermittent esotropia.

Treatment

● No treatment is needed. Parents can be reassured that most children will outgrow the appearance of crossing.

Prognosis

● As the child grows, the bridge of the nose becomes more prominent and displaces the epicanthal folds, and the medial sclera becomes proportional to the amount visible on the lateral aspect of the eye. Parents should be cautioned that children with pseudoesotropia, like any child, can develop true strabismus later in life. Therefore, if a change in appearance occurs, a repeat evaluation may be warranted.

CONGENITAL (INFANTILE) ESOTROPIA

Epidemiology and Etiology

- The cause of congenital esotropia is unknown. Theories include both a primary defect in sensory development of the brain that leads to abnormal alignment and a primary "motor" theory in which the ocular misalignment is the primary abnormality, which then leads to a secondary disruption of binocular vision. It is likely that both causes exist and may also be equally responsible for the development of the disorder in many children.

- The incidence of congenital esotropia is approximately 1 in 1000 children.

Signs and Symptoms

- Few children who are eventually diagnosed with this disorder are actually born with an esotropia. Although parents often give a history of their child's eyes crossing since birth, the crossing is rarely seen in the newborn nursery and is generally not observed during the first few weeks of life.

- The diagnosis is generally made when an infant presents before 6 months of age with a large ($\geq$30 prism diopter), constant esotropia, full abduction, a normal level of hyperopia, and no underlying ophthalmic disorder that could lead to vision loss and a secondary strabismus (Fig. 11-2). Children with congenital esotropia often appear to exhibit an apparent abduction deficit. This pseudoparesis is usually secondary to the presence of cross fixation. If the child has equal vision, he or she will have no need to abduct either eye. The child will use the adducted, or crossed, eye to look to the opposite field of gaze. In this case, he or she will show a bilateral

pseudoparesis of abduction. If amblyopia is present, only the better-seeing eye will cross fixate, making the amblyopic eye appear to have an abduction weakness. To differentiate between a true abducens paralysis and a pseudoparalysis, a doll's head maneuver can be used or abduction can be examined after the infant has worn a patch over one eye for a period of time.

Differential Diagnosis

- Pseudoesotropia
- Duane retraction syndrome
- Möbius syndrome
- Congenital sixth nerve palsy
- Early-onset accommodative esotropia
- Sensory esotropia
- Esotropia in the neurologically impaired

Diagnostic Evaluation

- All children with suspected congenital esotropia should undergo a complete examination, including a dilated funduscopic evaluation and cycloplegic refraction to rule out possible early-onset accommodative esotropia or a secondary strabismus (Fig. 11-3).

- Amblyopia can be diagnosed by looking for a fixation preference.

- If an accommodative component to the crossing is considered to be a possibility, the child should be given the full cycloplegic refraction and reevaluated to look for any effect on the crossing.

Treatment

- The treatment for congenital esotropia consists of strabismus surgery. Surgery is performed after any associated amblyopia, if present, is treated. It is important to treat amblyopia before surgery. It is much easier to follow the progress of amblyopia in a preverbal child while his or her eyes are crossed. In addition, parental compliance with amblyopia treatment tends to be much lower after the eyes are straightened and appear "normal."

- The primary goal of treatment in congenital esotropia is to eliminate or reduce the deviation as much as possible. Ideally, this results in normal visual acuity in each eye, straight-looking eyes, and the development of binocular vision.

Prognosis

- Children with congenital esotropia do not develop normal (bifoveal) binocular vision. Successful treatment provides the opportunity to develop some degree of binocular vision (monofixation syndrome), which allows the development of motor fusion and helps to keep their eyes aligned.

- Even with successful initial treatment, many children with a history of congenital esotropia may redevelop strabismus or amblyopia and therefore need to be monitored closely during the visually immature period of life.

- Recurrent horizontal strabismus is common as are vertical deviations. These may develop months or years after the initial surgery has been performed. The two most common forms of vertical deviations to develop are inferior oblique muscle overaction (IOOA) and dissociated vertical deviation (DVD).

REFERENCES

Archer SM, Sondhi N, Helveston EM. Strabismus in infancy. *Ophthalmology.* 1989;96:133.

Arthur BW, Smith JT, Scott WE. Long-term stability of alignment in the monofixation syndrome. *J Pediatr Ophthalmol Strabismus.* 1989;26:224.

Birch E, Stager D, Wright K, et al. The natural history of infantile esotropia during the first six months of life. *J AAPOS.* 1998;2:325–328.

Birch EE, Stager DR, Everett ME. Random dot stereoacuity following surgical correction of infantile esotropia. *J Pediatr Ophthalmol Strabismus.* 1995;32:231.

Ing M, Costenbader FD, Parks MM, et al. Early surgery for congenital esotropia. *Am J Ophthalmol.* 1966;62:1419.

Parks MM. The monofixation syndrome. *Trans Am Ophthalmol Soc.* 1969;67:609.

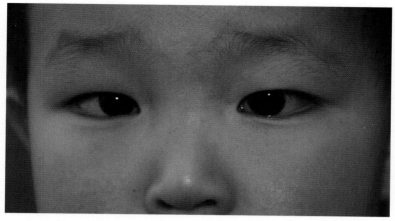

FIGURE 11-1. Pseudoesotropia. Pseudoesotropia caused by a wide nasal bridge and epicanthal folds. Note that the child is looking slightly to the left which also accentuates the false appearance that there is less sclera in the right eye.

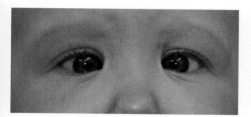

FIGURE 11-2. Congenital (infantile) esotropia. (From Nelson LB, Olitsky SE. *A Color Handbook of Pediatric Clinical Ophthalmology*. London, England: Manson Publishing; 2011.)

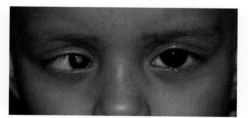

FIGURE 11-3. Sensory esotropia. Sensory esotropia secondary to a congenital cataract in the right eye.

INFERIOR OBLIQUE OVERACTION

Epidemiology and Etiology

● Inferior oblique overaction occurs in a primary and secondary form. Most patients with primary IOOA have a history of congenital esotropia, but it may occur in association with other forms of strabismus as well. Up to 80% of patients with a history of congenital esotropia may develop IOOA. Secondary IOOA occurs in patients with superior oblique palsy.

Signs and Symptoms

● IOOA results in elevation of the involved eye as it moves nasally (Fig. 11-4).

Differential Diagnosis

● DVD

● Duane syndrome with upshoot

Diagnostic Evaluation

● The amount of overaction is evaluated in the field of action of the inferior oblique muscle in question. IOOA can be classified as grades I to IV. Grade I represents 1 mm of higher elevation of the adducting eye in gaze up and to the side. Grade IV indicates 4 mm of higher elevation. These differences in elevation between the two eyes are measured from the 6-o'clock position on each limbus. A measurement of the degree of adduction that is required to elicit the overaction is also helpful when considering treatment.

Treatment

● IOOA can be treated surgically. The thresholds for surgery for IOOA are different, depending on whether weakening the inferior oblique is the only surgery being contemplated or whether weakening the inferior oblique in conjunction with horizontal strabismus surgery is being considered. If the inferior obliques alone are weakened, there should be a significant overaction present to justify surgery. If horizontal surgery is being performed, smaller grades of inferior oblique overaction may be corrected at the same time. Inferior oblique recession, myotomy, myectomy, or denervation and extirpation can be performed to weaken the action of the inferior oblique.

● Anterior transposition of the inferior oblique can also be performed to limit the elevation of the eye and may be the treatment of choice when both IOOA and DVD occur together.

Prognosis

● Surgery is generally successful in improving the overacting inferior oblique muscle. Care must be taken to not miss any fibers of the muscle at the time of surgery.

REFERENCES

Parks MM. A study of the weakening surgical procedure for eliminating overaction of the inferior oblique. *Am J Ophthalmol.* 1972;73:107.

Stager DR. Costenbader lecture. Anatomy and surgery of the inferior oblique muscle: recent findings. *J AAPOS.* 2001;5:203–208.

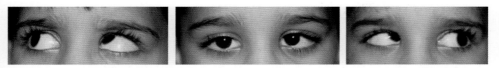

FIGURE 11-4. Inferior oblique overaction. Inferior oblique overaction in both eyes. Note the elevation of each eye in adduction.

DISSOCIATED VERTICAL DEVIATION

Epidemiology and Etiology

● Most patients with DVD have a history of congenital esotropia, but it may occur in association with other forms of strabismus as well.

● Up to 90% of patients with a history of congenital esotropia may develop DVD.

● DVD appears to be a time-related phenomenon and is not related to successful initial surgery or the development of binocular vision.

Signs and Symptoms

● DVD consists of a slow upward deviation of one or alternate eyes (**Fig. 11-5**). Excyclotorsion can often be demonstrated on upward drifting of the eye and incyclotorsion on downward motion.

● DVD may be latent, detected only when the involved eye is covered, or manifest, occurring intermittently or constantly. It can be differentiated from a true vertical deviation because no corresponding hypotropia occurs in the other eye on cover testing.

Differential Diagnosis

● Inferior oblique overaction

● Hypertropia

Diagnostic Evaluation

● DVD can be estimated by using the Hirschberg and Krimsky methods or the prism cover test. A base-down prism is placed over the involved eye. The strength of the prism is adjusted until no movement occurs as the cover is shifted from the involved to the fixating eye. Because prism cover measurement is difficult and may be inaccurate, DVD can also be estimated using a semiquantitative grading scale (1 to 4+).

Treatment

● If amblyopia exists, improvement in vision may improve fusional control and decrease how frequently the deviation is manifest.

● If DVD is entirely latent, detected on cover testing only, surgery is not indicated. If it is intermittent, surgery is determined by the size and frequency of the deviation as well as the patient's concern regarding its appearance. Surgical treatment for DVD includes recession of the superior rectus and recession of the superior rectus combined with a posterior fixation suture and anterior transposition of the inferior oblique (preferred if IOOA coexists).

Prognosis

● It is often not possible to completely eliminate DVD. The goal of treatment is to reduce the magnitude of the deviation enough that it is not noticeable when it is manifest.

REFERENCES

Bacal DA, Nelson LB. Anterior transposition of the inferior oblique muscle for both dissociated vertical deviation and/or inferior oblique overaction: results of 94 procedures in 55 patients. *Binocular Vision Eye Muscle Surg.* 1992;7:219.

Christoff A, Raab EL, Guyton DL, et al. DVD—a conceptual, clinical, and surgical overview. *J AAPOS.* 2014;18:378–384.

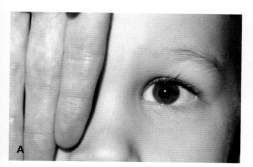
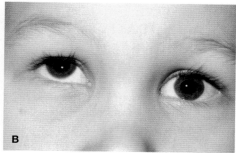

FIGURE 11-5. Dissociated vertical deviation. A. Right eye occluded. **B.** Dissociated vertical deviation manifest after occlusion. (Courtesy of Alex Levin, MD.)

REFRACTIVE ACCOMMODATIVE ESOTROPIA

Epidemiology and Etiology

- The mechanism of refractive accommodative esotropia involves three factors: uncorrected hyperopia, accommodative convergence, and insufficient fusional divergence. When an individual exerts a given amount of accommodation, a specific amount of convergence (accommodative convergence) is associated with it. An uncorrected hyperopia must exert excessive accommodation to clear a blurred retinal image. This in turn stimulates excessive convergence. If the amplitude of fusional divergence is sufficient to correct the excess convergence, no esotropia will result. However, if the fusional divergence amplitudes are inadequate or motor fusion is altered by some sensory obstacle, an esotropia will result.

Signs and Symptoms

- Refractive accommodative esotropia usually occurs in a child between 2 and 3 years of age with a history of acquired intermittent or constant esotropia. Occasionally, children who are 1 year of age or younger present with accommodative esotropia.

- The refraction of patients with refractive accommodative esotropia averages +4.75 diopters. The angle of esodeviation is the same when measured at distance and near fixation and is usually moderate in magnitude, ranging between 20 and 40 prism diopters. Amblyopia is common, especially when the esodeviation has become increasingly constant.

Differential Diagnosis

- Congenital esotropia
- Nonaccommodative esotropia
- Nonrefractive accommodative esotropia

Diagnostic Evaluation

- A complete examination should be performed, including a cycloplegic refraction.

Treatment

- The full hyperopic correction, determined by cycloplegic refraction, should be prescribed.

Prognosis

- Most children will maintain straight eyes while wearing their glasses (Fig. 11-6). Some children may show an increase in their hyperopia, which can lead to a recurrent crossing. A nonaccommodative esotropia may develop in a small percentage of children. Patients with relatively smaller levels of hyperopia may eventually outgrow their need for glasses as their hyperopic refractive error lessens with age.

REFERENCES

Coats DK, Avilla CW, Paysse EA, et al. Early-onset refractive accommodative esotropia. *J AAPOS*. 1998;2:275–278.

Raab EL. Etiologic factors in accommodative esodeviation. *Trans Am Ophthalmol Soc.* 1982;80:657.

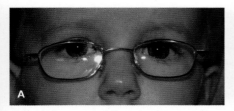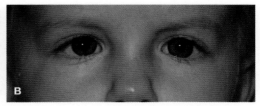

FIGURE 11-6. **Refractive accommodative esotropia.** **A.** With the appropriate hyperopic glasses, the eyes are straight. **B.** Without glasses, there is an esotropia of 25 prism diopters.

NONREFRACTIVE ACCOMMODATIVE ESOTROPIA

Epidemiology and Etiology

● Children with nonrefractive accommodative esotropia usually present between 2 and 3 years of age with an esodeviation that is greater at near than at distance fixation. The refractive error in this condition may be hyperopic or myopic, although the average refraction is +2.25 diopters.

● In nonrefractive accommodative esotropia, there is a high accommodative convergence–to–accommodation (AC:A) ratio: The effort to accommodate elicits an abnormally high accommodative convergence response.

Signs and Symptoms

● Some parents notice the crossing that only takes place at near fixation.

● There are a number of ways of measuring the AC:A ratio. Most clinicians prefer to assess the ratio using the distance–near comparison. The AC:A relationship is derived by simply comparing the distance and near deviation. If the near measurement in a patient with esotropia is greater than 10 prism diopters, the AC:A ratio is considered to be abnormally high.

Differential Diagnosis

● Refractive accommodative esotropia

Diagnostic Evaluation

● A complete examination, including a measurement of the esotropia at both distance and near fixation as well as a cycloplegic refraction, should be performed.

Treatment

● Treatment often involves the use of bifocal lenses to eliminate the accommodative effort required for near work. The bifocal is usually prescribed as an executive-type lens that bisects the pupil.

● Another treatment option is strabismus surgery. Some patients may be followed because those with good alignment at distance usually develop normal vision.

Prognosis

● Many patients show a normalization of their AC:A ratio over time.

● Some patients decompensate and develop a nonaccommodative component that may require surgery. The risk of decompensation appears to be related to the magnitude of the distance–near disparity of the crossing.

REFERENCES

Kushner BJ. Fifteen-year outcome of surgery for the near angle in patients with accommodative esotropia and a high accommodative convergence to accommodation ratio. *Arch Ophthalmol.* 2001;119:1150–1153.

Ludwig IH, Parks MM, Getson PR. Long-term results of bifocal therapy for accommodative esotropia. *J Pediatr Ophthalmol Strabismus.* 1989;26:264.

Pratt-Johnson JA, Tillson G. The management of esotropia with high AC/A ratio (convergence excess). *J Pediatr Ophthalmol Strabismus.* 1985;22:238.

Whitman MC, MacNeill K, Hunter DG. Bifocals fail to improve stereopsis outcomes in high AC/A accommodative esotropia. *Ophthalmology.* 2016;123:690–696.

NONACCOMMODATIVE OR PARTIALLY ACCOMMODATIVE ESOTROPIA

Epidemiology and Etiology

● Refractive or nonrefractive accommodative esotropias do not always occur in their "pure" forms. Some patients may show no response to correction of their hyperopia. Other patients may have a significant reduction in esodeviation when given glasses, but a residual esodeviation persists despite full hyperopic correction. Still others may show an initial good response only to develop a crossing that can no longer be completely corrected with glasses. The crossing not corrected with the glasses is the nonaccommodative portion. This condition commonly occurs when there is a delay of months between the onset of accommodative esotropia and antiaccommodative treatment.

Signs and Symptoms

● Patients with nonaccommodative esotropia have little or no hyperopia. They may also have a level of hyperopia that does not appear compatible with the degree of crossing.

● Patients with a partial accommodative esotropia appear to have a level of hyperopia that will correct their crossing. However, they do not demonstrate a resolution of their crossing when wearing their glasses.

Differential Diagnosis

● Congenital esotropia

● Accommodative esotropia

Diagnostic Evaluation

● A complete examination with cycloplegic refraction should be performed. If a significant level of hyperopia exists, the patient should be prescribed the full hyperopic correction and return after wearing glasses for a period of time.

Treatment

● If the nonaccommodative component of the crossing is large enough to prevent the development of binocular vision, strabismus surgery should be considered. Some surgeons will not opt for surgery if the crossing is small and not easily noticed.

Prognosis

● Patients with small levels of hyperopia may be able to discontinue wearing their glasses. Recurrent strabismus is possible in these patients, who often have abnormal binocular vision even after successful treatment.

CONGENITAL EXOTROPIA

Epidemiology and Etiology

● Congenital exotropia behaves in a very similar fashion to congenital esotropia. It typically occurs early in life and presents with a large, constant out-turning. Congenital exotropia may be associated with neurologic disease or abnormalities of the bony orbit, as in Crouzon syndrome.

Signs and Symptoms

● Patients with congenital exotropia often appear to have decreased adduction on side gaze; with gaze right or left, the abducting eye fixates, whereas the opposite eye approaches midline and stops. This is similar to the cross fixation found in children with congenital esotropia. Occlusion or the doll's head maneuver will demonstrate that good adduction is possible.

● Amblyopia is not common because these children typically alternate fixation. The refractive error is similar to that of the general population.

Differential Diagnosis

● Early-onset intermittent exotropia

● Third cranial nerve palsy

● Bilateral intranuclear ophthalmoplegia

Diagnostic Evaluation

● A complete examination should be performed.

● Other signs of a cranial nerve palsy (ptosis, decreased motility) should be eliminated.

Treatment

● Patients with congenital constant exotropia are operated on early in life in the same manner as patients with congenital esotropia.

Prognosis

● Similar to patients with congenital esotropia, early surgery in these patients can lead to gross binocular vision but not bifoveal fixation.

● These patients also tend to develop DVD and IOOA and should be followed closely for the development of these associated motility disturbances.

REFERENCE

Hunter DG, Kelly JB, Buffenn AN, et al. Long-term outcome of uncomplicated infantile exotropia. *J AAPOS.* 2001;5:352–356.

INTERMITTENT EXOTROPIA

Epidemiology and Etiology

● Intermittent exotropia is the most common exodeviation in childhood.

● The etiology of intermittent exotropia is unknown but probably results from a combination of mechanical and innervational factors.

Signs and Symptoms

● The age of onset of intermittent exotropia varies but is often between 6 months and 4 years.

● It is characterized by outward drifting of one eye, which usually occurs when a child is fixating at a distance (**Fig. 11-7**). The deviation is generally more frequent with fatigue or illness. Exposure to bright light may cause reflex closure of the exotropic eye.

● Because the deviation generally begins with distance fixation and is only seen when the child is tired, it is often not seen when the child is examined by a primary medical doctor at close distance or during a well-child visit.

Differential Diagnosis

● Congenital exotropia

Diagnostic Evaluation

● A complete evaluation should be performed. Motility measurements at both distance and near fixation should be completed. A qualitative measurement of the control of the strabismus should be noted.

Treatment

● Any coexistent amblyopia should be treated. Significant refractive errors should be corrected. Some ophthalmologists use medical treatments to avoid surgery in some patients. These nonsurgical treatments include part-time occlusion, orthoptic therapy, and over-minus lens therapy. Most patients eventually require strabismus surgery when the deviation becomes manifest frequently.

Prognosis

● Surgery is successful in aligning most patients' eyes. Some patients will redevelop strabismus and may require more surgery.

REFERENCES

Kushner BJ. Exotropic deviations: a functional classification and approach to treatment. *Am Orthoptic J.* 1988;38:81–93.
Pediatric Eye Disease Investigator Group. A randomized trial comparing part-time patching with observation for intermittent exotropia in children 12 to 35 months of age. *Ophthalmology.* 2015:1718–1725.

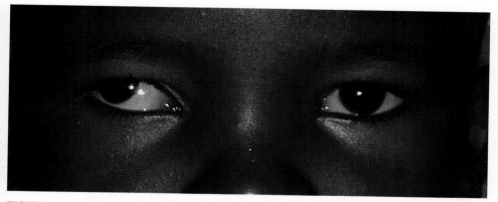

FIGURE 11-7. Intermittent exotropia. Intermittent exotropia demonstrating manifest exotropia at distance fixation.

A AND V PATTERN STRABISMUS

Epidemiology and Etiology

- A and V patterns are manifested by a horizontal change of alignment as the eyes move from the primary position to midline upgaze or downgaze.

- A number of different theories have evolved to explain the etiology of A and V patterns. There is no universal agreement of their cause at this time.

- Oblique muscle dysfunction is often seen in the setting of A and V pattern strabismus (Figs. 11-8 and 11-9). The oblique muscles have secondary abducting action. Therefore, when the superior obliques are overacting, they may cause an A pattern; when the inferior obliques are overacting or the superior obliques are underacting, a V pattern often results. However, A and V patterns frequently exist in the absence of demonstrable oblique dysfunction.

Signs and Symptoms

- Esotropia with V pattern increases in downgaze and decreases in upgaze. The deviation in V exotropia increases in upgaze and decreases in downgaze.

- In A esotropia, the deviation increases in upgaze and decreases in downgaze.

- In A exotropia, the deviation increases in downgaze and decreases in upgaze.

- Anomalous head posture is common in patients with A and V patterns.

- Patients with A esotropia and V exotropia and fusion in downgaze may develop a chin-up position. Conversely, V esotropia and A exotropia may cause chin depression.

Differential Diagnosis

- A and V pattern strabismus should be looked for in patients with compensatory chin-up or chin-down strabismus.

- Restrictive or paralytic strabismus may also present with abnormal head postures.

- Brown syndrome may manifest a V pattern.

Diagnostic Evaluation

- The A and V patterns are demonstrated by measuring a deviation in primary position and in approximately 25 degrees of upgaze and downgaze while the patient fixates on a distant object.

- An A pattern is said to exist if divergence increases in downgaze by 10 or more prism diopters.

- A V pattern signifies an increase in divergence of 15 or more prism diopters in upgaze. The smaller amount of change required to make a diagnosis of an A pattern is caused by the greater effect of the downgaze deviation on reading and other near tasks.

Treatment

- Patients with torticollis may benefit from treatment. Patients with large patterns often have significant oblique dysfunction. Treatment of the oblique dysfunction is usually needed to treat these large patterns. However, superior oblique weakening should be done with extreme caution in patients with A pattern strabismus and good binocular function because an asymmetric result can lead to permanent torsional diplopia. In patients without oblique dysfunction, vertically moving or offsetting the horizontal rectus muscle weakens the action of that muscle when the eye is moved in the direction of the offsetting. For example, if the medial rectus muscles are moved up one-half tendon width, their horizontal action further decreases in upgaze. Therefore, moving the medial rectus toward the apex of an A and V pattern or moving the lateral rectus muscle toward the open end of the A or V is appropriate for correcting the incomitant deviation. This is true regardless of whether recession or resection is performed.

The tendon is generally moved up or down half of its insertion width.

Prognosis

● Surgery is generally effective in collapsing the pattern and decreasing or eliminating the associated head posture when present.

REFERENCES

Knapp P. Vertically incomitant horizontal strabismus: the so called A and V syndrome. *Trans Am Ophthalmol Soc.* 1959;57:666–698.

Scott WE, Drummond GT, Keech RV. Vertical offsets of horizontal recti muscles in the management of A and V pattern strabismus. *Aust N Z J Ophthalmol.* 1989;17:281.

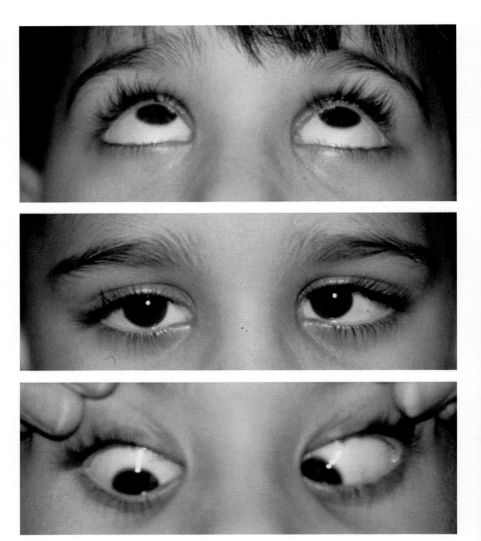

FIGURE 11-8. V pattern esotropia. The esotropia increases in straight downgaze and decreases in straight upgaze.

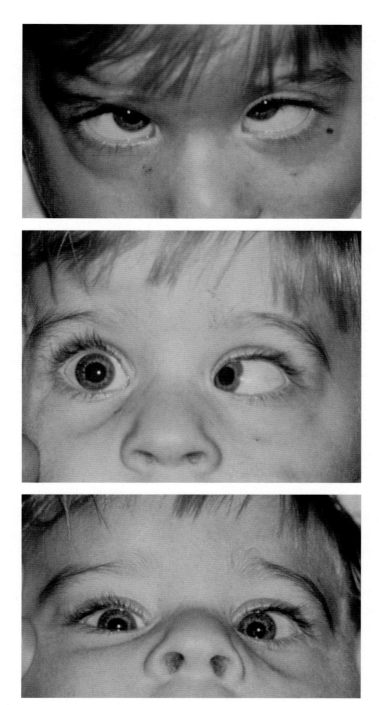

FIGURE 11-9. A pattern esotropia. The esotropia increases in straight upgaze and decreases in straight downgaze.

THIRD NERVE PALSY

Epidemiology and Etiology

- In children, third nerve palsies are usually congenital. The congenital form is often associated with a developmental anomaly or birth trauma. Acquired third nerve palsies can be an ominous sign and may indicate a neurologic abnormality, such as an intracranial neoplasm or an aneurysm. Other less serious causes include an inflammatory or infectious lesion, head trauma, postviral syndromes, and migraines.

Signs and Symptoms

- A third nerve palsy, whether congenital or acquired, usually results in an exotropia and a hypotropia of the affected eye, as well as complete or partial ptosis of the upper eyelid (Fig. 11-10A). This characteristic strabismus results from the action of the normal, unopposed muscles, the lateral rectus muscle and the superior oblique muscle. If the internal branch of the third nerve is involved, pupillary dilation may be noted as well. Adduction, elevation, and depression are usually limited (Fig. 11-10B).

- In congenital and traumatic cases of third nerve palsy, a misdirection of regenerating nerve fibers may develop, referred to as *aberrant regeneration*. This results in anomalous and paradoxical eyelid, eye, and pupil movement, such as elevation of the eyelid, constriction of the pupil, or depression of the globe on attempted adduction.

Differential Diagnosis

- Congenital exotropia

- Congenital fibrosis of the extraocular muscles (CFEOM)

Diagnostic Evaluation

- Diagnosis is based on the characteristic exotropia and hypotropia with associated limitation in adduction and vertical movements of the eye.

- Pupillary involvement is an especially important sign because it may indicate an expanding intracranial aneurysm and need for emergent neurologic evaluation and treatment.

- Patients with acquired third nerve palsy should have a neurologic evaluation, including neuroimaging when indicated.

Treatment

- Initial treatment for patients with acquired third nerve palsy involves relief of diplopia. If there is complete third nerve palsy, the associated complete ptosis will cover the pupil and prevent diplopia. However, in partial third nerve palsy, the eyelid may not cover the pupillary space, so diplopia may remain a problem. Occlusion therapy is then the best solution for the diplopia. In children young enough to develop amblyopia, the patch should be alternated, so the affected eye will continue to develop normal vision.

- Surgery to correct acquired third nerve palsy should be postponed for several months after the onset of the condition when possible. If the ptosis is complete and the eyelid cannot open, early ptosis surgery may be needed in younger children to prevent the development of amblyopia. In a complete third nerve palsy, the motility of the globe is severely limited because only the lateral rectus and superior oblique muscles are functional. Surgical options include lateral rectus recession, superior oblique weakening or transposition, splitting of the lateral rectus with transposition adjacent to the medial rectus, and fixation of the globe to the orbital wall with a nonabsorbable suture or fascia lata.

Prognosis

- The goal of surgical intervention is to use the two remaining functional muscles in such a way as to achieve a straight-ahead eye with only limited movement of the globe. This goal should be carefully explained to the patient and the parents to avoid unrealistic postoperative expectations.

REFERENCES

Gokyigit B, Akar S, Satana B, Demirok A, Yilmaz OF. Medial transposition of a split lateral rectus muscle for complete oculomotor nerve palsy. *J AAPOS.* 2013;17:402–410.

Keane JR. Third nerve palsy: analysis of 1400 personally-examined inpatients. *Can J Neurol Sci.* 2010;37:662–670.

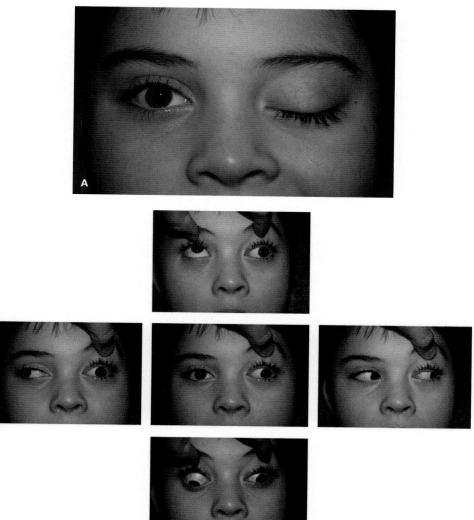

FIGURE 11-10. Third nerve palsy. A and **B.** Third nerve palsy. (From Nelson LB, Olitsky SE. *A Color Handbook of Pediatric Clinical Ophthalmology.* London, England: Manson Publishing; 2011.)

FOURTH NERVE PALSY

Epidemiology and Etiology

• Fourth nerve palsy is the most common cause of an isolated cyclovertical muscle palsy. Paresis of the fourth nerve can be congenital or acquired. Closed-head trauma is the most common cause of acquired fourth nerve palsy, and other causes include cerebrovascular accident, diabetes, brain tumor, ethmoiditis, or mastoiditis.

Signs and Symptoms

• Patients with unilateral fourth nerve palsy often present with torticollis to reduce diplopia. This usually consists of a head tilt to the side of the nonparetic eye, a face turn to the contralateral side, and a small chin-down head posture. Patients with a bilateral palsy usually place their heads in a chin-down position.

• The absence of a head tilt in a preverbal child should raise the suspicion of amblyopia.

• Facial asymmetry has been associated with congenital superior oblique palsy and is typically manifested by midfacial hemihypoplasia on the dependent side opposite the affected superior oblique. The nose deviates toward the hypoplastic side, and the mouth slants so that it approximates a horizontal orientation despite the torticollis.

Differential Diagnosis

• Any vertical strabismus that leads to a hypertropia

Diagnostic Evaluation

• To evaluate a suspected fourth nerve palsy, a three-step test should be performed. A patient with a fourth nerve palsy will demonstrate a hypertropia that is worse when looking to the contralateral side and when the head is tilted to the ipsilateral side of the affected eye (Fig. 11-11). The three-step test is most useful when the strabismus is acute and may miss some cases of radiologically confirmed superior oblique palsies.

• When a patient presents with a new onset of diplopia secondary to a fourth nerve palsy, it is important to determine if the palsy has only recently developed or if it represents a congenital disorder that has decompensated. Several features may help to determine the acuteness of the deviation. A patient with a congenital superior oblique palsy will often have large vertical fusional amplitudes and a long-standing head tilt that can be documented in old photographs. Facial asymmetry may be present.

• In patients with a fourth nerve palsy, bilateral involvement should be excluded. Signs of bilateral fourth nerve palsy include hypertropia that alternates in right and left gaze and in right and left head tilt, a V pattern esotropia, and a large degree of excyclotorsion on either double Maddox rod testing or funduscopic evaluation.

Treatment

• Except for an occasional patient with a fairly comitant vertical deviation of 10 prism diopters or less (when prism may be tolerated), most cases of superior oblique palsy require surgery. In general, surgery for superior oblique palsies should be directed to those muscles whose greatest action is in the field when the vertical deviation is the largest. Surgical options include superior oblique tuck, inferior oblique weakening, ipsilateral superior rectus recession or contralateral inferior rectus recession, or various combinations of these procedures.

Prognosis

● Surgical treatment is helpful in reducing or eliminating the abnormal head posture, normalizing ocular rotations, and enlarging the area of single binocular vision in most patients.

REFERENCES

Manchandia AM, Demer JL. Sensitivity of the three-step test in diagnosis of superior oblique palsy. *J AAPOS.* 2014;18:567–571.

Parks MM. Isolated cyclovertical muscle palsy. *Arch Ophthalmol.* 1958;60:1027.

Wilson ME, Hoxie J. Facial asymmetry in superior oblique muscle palsy. *J Pediatr Ophthalmol Strabismus.* 1993;30:315.

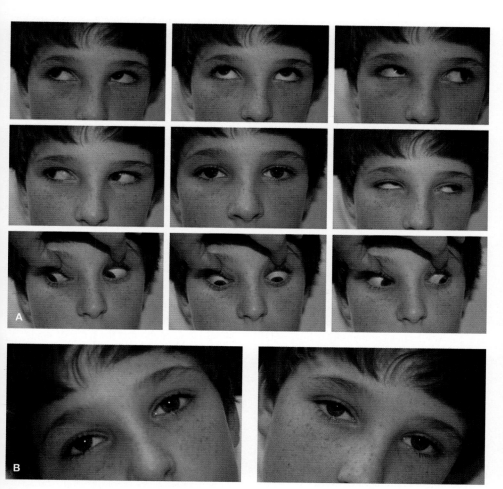

FIGURE 11-11. Fourth nerve palsy. A and **B.** Fourth nerve palsy.

SIXTH NERVE PALSY

Epidemiology and Etiology

- Sixth nerve palsies can be congenital or acquired (Fig. 11-12). Congenital sixth nerve palsies are rare. Acquired sixth nerve palsy is more common.

- The sixth nerve has a long intracranial course, and there are three anatomic areas where the sixth nerve is most susceptible to injury: (1) as it exits from the pontomedullary junction, (2) at its penetration of the dura (Dorello canal), and (3) within the cavernous sinus.

- Trauma is probably the most common cause of acquired sixth nerve palsy. Other causes include neoplastic, inflammatory, vascular, and postviral. Acquired bilateral sixth nerve palsy is usually a manifestation of a serious intracranial abnormality or an increase in intracranial pressure (ICP).

Signs and Symptoms

- Patients with acute sixth nerve palsy usually present with diplopia. If the palsy is unilateral, double vision may be avoided by adopting a compensatory head posture with the eyes in the lateral gaze position away from the palsied eye; this results in a compensatory horizontal face turn toward the palsied eye.

Differential Diagnosis

- Congenital esotropia
- Duane syndrome
- Möbius syndrome

Diagnostic Evaluation

- A complete examination should be performed, and signs of increased ICP (papilledema) should be sought. Neurologic consultation and neuroimaging should be considered for most patients. A lumbar puncture may be needed to document increased ICP.

- Most patients with suspected congenital sixth nerve palsy have congenital esotropia with cross fixation of one or both eyes. It is important to identify these patients to avoid unnecessary diagnostic procedures.

Treatment

- Initial treatment may consist of occlusion to eliminate diplopia. Children with significant hyperopia should be given glasses to avoid the development of an accommodative esotropia. If the deviation does not improve over time, surgery may be necessary.

- If there is lateral rectus function, a unilateral medial rectus recession combined with a lateral rectus resection can be performed.

- If little or no function of the lateral rectus exists, a transposition procedure may be needed.

Prognosis

- Many patients can be given single vision with or without a small face turn. Patients should understand that the range of single binocular vision may be limited; this is especially true in bilateral cases.

REFERENCES

Brooks SE, Olitsky SE, deB Ribeiro G. Augmented Hummelsheim procedure for paralytic strabismus. *J Pediatr Ophthalmol Strabismus.* 2000;37:189–195.

Holmes JM, Beck RW, Kip KE, et al. Botulinum toxin treatment versus conservative management in acute traumatic sixth nerve palsy or paresis. *J AAPOS.* 2000;4:145–149.

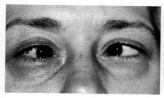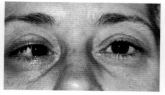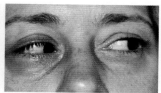

FIGURE 11-12. **Sixth nerve palsy.**

DUANE SYNDROME

Epidemiology and Etiology

• Duane syndrome is found in approximately 1% of individuals with strabismus. It occurs more frequently in the left eye than in the right and in females more than in males.

• Bilateral involvement is less frequent than unilateral occurrence (**Fig. 11-13**).

• Although Duane syndrome has been well described clinically, the etiology remains unclear. Various theories include structural and innervational anomalies of the extraocular muscles as well as absence or hypoplasia of the sixth nerve nucleus.

• Up- and downshoots that may be seen in Duane syndrome may occur because of coinnervation of the horizontal and vertical rectus muscles or slippage of the lateral rectus muscle above or below the eye, commonly referred to as a "leash phenomenon."

Signs and Symptoms

• The most characteristic clinical findings in Duane syndrome include an absence of abduction of an eye with slight limitation of adduction, retraction of the globe in attempted adduction, and up- and downshooting or both in adduction. Classically, Duane syndrome has been grouped into three types:

  ▪ Type I: marked limitation or complete absence of abduction; normal or only slightly restricted adduction

  ▪ Type II: limitation or absence of adduction with exotropia of the affected eye; normal or slightly limited abduction

  ▪ Type III: severe limitation of both abduction and adduction

• Other ocular or systemic anomalies are commonly seen in patients with Duane syndrome. Ocular anomalies may include dysplasia of the iris stroma, pupillary anomalies, cataracts, heterochromia, Marcus Gunn jaw winking, coloboma, crocodile tears, and microphthalmos. The systemic anomalies include Goldenhar syndrome; dystrophic defects such as Klippel-Feil syndrome; cervical spina bifida; cleft palate; facial anomalies; perceptive deafness; malformations of the external ear; and anomalies of the limbs, feet, and hands.

Differential Diagnosis

• Sixth nerve palsy
• Congenital esotropia
• Exotropia

Diagnostic Evaluation

• The disorder most commonly confused with Duane syndrome is sixth nerve palsy. Patients with a sixth nerve palsy generally have a much larger deviation in primary position than patients with Duane syndrome given the magnitude of the abduction deficit. In addition, an exotropia can usually be found in gaze to the opposite side in patients with Duane syndrome and does not occur in sixth nerve palsies.

Treatment

• Before surgery is contemplated, coexisting significant refractive errors, anisometropia, and amblyopia should be treated. Indications for surgery include a significant deviation in primary position, an anomalous head position, a large up- or downshoot, or retraction of the globe that is cosmetically intolerable.

• Surgery usually involves recession of the medial or lateral rectus for patients with esotropia of exotropia. Some surgeons prefer transposition surgery. The medial rectus of the involved eye is usually tight, and forced duction testing results are often positive because of the contracture of the muscle.

• Resection of the ipsilateral lateral rectus should almost never be performed because it will increase retraction of the globe in adduction. If an up- or downshoot of the eye occurs, surgical options include recessing a stiff, fibrotic lateral rectus muscle, performing a Y splitting of the muscle, or placement of a posterior fixation suture to reduce the leash effect when present.

● Patients who have a cosmetically noticeable retraction of the globe in attempted adduction may benefit from recession of both horizontal recti to reduce the co-contraction. This can be done in the absence of a deviation in primary gaze or adjusted to eliminate a deviation if present.

Prognosis

● Surgery can help to reduce or eliminate an associated torticollis. Few patients show improvement in abduction after surgery, and some patients undergoing medial rectus recession may have a decrease in adduction.

● In patients with significant co-contraction, large overcorrections can occur after medial rectus recession.

REFERENCE

Kekunnaya R, Kraft S, Rao VB, Velez FG, Sachdeva V, Hunter DG. Surgical management of strabismus in Duane retraction syndrome. *J AAPOS*. 2015;19:63–69.

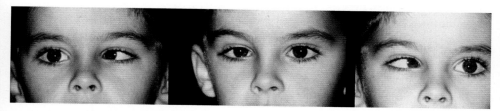

FIGURE 11-13. **Bilateral Duane syndrome.**

BROWN SYNDROME

Epidemiology and Etiology

- Brown syndrome may occur as a congenital or acquired defect and can be permanent, transient, or intermittent. Congenital Brown syndrome occurs because of an anomaly of the anterior sheath of the superior oblique tendon. The acquired form has been attributed to a variety of causes, including superior oblique surgery, scleral buckling bands, trauma, and after sinus surgery and inflammation in the trochlear region.

- Brown syndrome can be acquired in patients with juvenile or adult rheumatoid arthritis and represents a stenosing tenosynovitis of the trochlea that shares similar characteristics to inflammatory disorders that affect the tendons of the fingers.

Signs and Symptoms

- Brown syndrome is characterized by a deficiency of elevation in the adducting position. Improved elevation is usually apparent in the midline, with normal or near-normal elevation in abduction (Fig. 11-14). With lateral gaze in the opposite direction, the involved eye may depress in adduction. Exodeviation (V pattern) often occurs as the eyes are moved upward in the midline. Many patients are orthophoric in primary position.

- If a hypotropia is present, the patient may develop a compensatory face turn toward the opposite eye.

- In some cases, there is discomfort on attempted elevation in adduction, the patient may feel or even hear a click under the same circumstances, and there may be a palpable mass or tenderness in the trochlear region. A positive forced duction test result is the hallmark of Brown syndrome.

Differential Diagnosis

- Inferior oblique palsy
- Superior oblique overaction
- Monocular elevation deficiency (MED)

Diagnostic Evaluation

- Patients will often display a V pattern, which helps distinguish Brown syndrome from superior oblique overaction (A pattern).

- Forced duction testing should be performed; results are positive in individuals with Brown syndrome.

Treatment

- Treatment is generally reserved for patients with a compensatory head posture, a hypotropia in primary position, or a large downshoot in adduction.

- Surgical treatment consists of a weakening procedure of the superior oblique tendon, which may include partial or full tenotomy, superior oblique recession, or superior oblique spacer.

- Patients with Brown syndrome secondary to an inflammatory process may respond to corticosteroids or nonsteroidal anti-inflammatory agents given systemically as well as injection of corticosteroids into the trochlear region.

Prognosis

- Up to one-third of patients that undergo superior oblique tenotomy develop an iatrogenic superior oblique palsy that may require further surgery.

- Even with successful surgery, elevation in adduction may continue to be abnormal in some patients.

REFERENCES

Helveston EM, Merriam WW, Ellis FD, et al. The trochlea. A study of the anatomy and physiology. *Ophthalmology.* 1982;89(2):124–133.

Parks MM, Eustis HS. Simultaneous superior oblique tenotomy and inferior oblique recession in Brown's syndrome. *Ophthalmology.* 1987;94:1043.

Wright KW. Superior oblique silicone expander for Brown's syndrome and superior oblique overaction. *J Pediatr Ophthalmol Strabismus.* 1991;28:101.

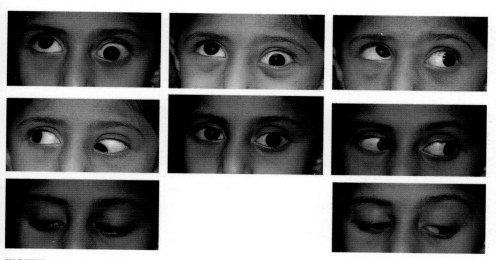

FIGURE 11-14. Acquired Brown syndrome.

MÖBIUS SYNDROME

Epidemiology and Etiology

- Möbius syndrome is a rare congenital disturbance consisting of varying involvement of facial and lateral gaze paresis.

- The etiology of Möbius syndrome is presently unknown. Theories to explain this condition include a mesodermal dysplasia involving musculature derived from the first and second branchial arches or a vascular theory with disruption of blood flow during embryogenesis.

Signs and Symptoms

- Möbius syndrome is characterized by a unilateral or bilateral inability to abduct the eyes. Although horizontal movements are usually lacking, vertical movements and convergence are intact.

- Esotropia is common in children with Möbius syndrome (**Fig. 11-15**).

- Unilateral or bilateral complete or incomplete facial palsy is usually observed during the first few weeks of life because of difficulty with sucking and feeding and incomplete closure of the eyelids during sleep. These patients typically have masklike faces with an inability to grin and wrinkle the forehead.

Differential Diagnosis

- Congenital esotropia
- Bilateral cranial nerve sixth palsy

Diagnostic Evaluation

- Similar to that in congenital esotropia. Patients show an abduction deficit and may be forced duction positive on testing in the operating room.

- Most patients carry a diagnosis before seeing an ophthalmologist. However, the presence of bilateral abduction deficit, typical facial appearance, and difficulty feeding should prompt a further evaluation with a geneticist if a diagnosis has not been made.

Treatment

- Strabismus surgery is usually required to align the eyes. Transposition surgery is preferred by some ophthalmologists.

Prognosis

- Alignment in primary position is possible in most patients.

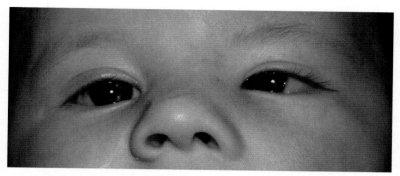

FIGURE 11-15. Möbius syndrome. (From Nelson LB, Olitsky SE. *A Color Handbook of Pediatric Clinical Ophthalmology*. London, England: Manson Publishing; 2011.)

MONOCULAR ELEVATION DEFICIENCY

Epidemiology and Etiology

● MED, formerly called double elevator palsy, suggests that both elevator muscles (the superior rectus and inferior oblique muscles) of one eye are weak, with a resultant inability or reduced ability to elevate the eye and a hypotropia in the primary position (Fig. 11-16). The term is generally used to describe diminished ocular elevation present in all fields of gaze.

● MED may be caused by innervational problems, restrictive conditions, or a combination of factors.

Signs and Symptoms

● Patients may present with a hypotropia or apparent ptosis. Some patients may develop a compensatory head posture with their chin in an upward position to maintain binocular vision.

● There is an inability to elevate the eye in all fields of gaze.

● In patients with restriction of upgaze, there may be an accentuated lower eyelid fold associated with inferior rectus restriction. This fold becomes more prominent with attempted upgaze.

Differential Diagnosis

● Brown syndrome

● Thyroid-related strabismus with inferior rectus muscle restriction

● Orbital floor fracture with entrapment of the inferior rectus muscle

Diagnostic Evaluation

● The presence of a true ptosis should be ruled out by forcing the patient to fixate with the involved eye. In cases of pseudoptosis caused by the ipsilateral hypotropia, the ptosis will disappear when the eye is brought to midline.

● Forced duction testing is needed to eliminate a restricted inferior rectus muscle as the cause of the MED.

Treatment

● In cases of inferior rectus muscle restriction, the involved muscle should be recessed. When no restriction is present, a transposition procedure (Knapp procedure) is usually required.

Prognosis

● Alignment in primary position and reduction of the abnormal head posture are the goals of treatment.

● Elevation is not usually improved in cases involving a weakness of the elevator muscles.

REFERENCES

Metz HS. Double elevator palsy. *Arch Ophthalmol.* 1979;97:901.
Scott WE, Jackson OB. Double elevator palsy: the significance of inferior rectus restriction. *Am Orthop J.* 1977;27:5.

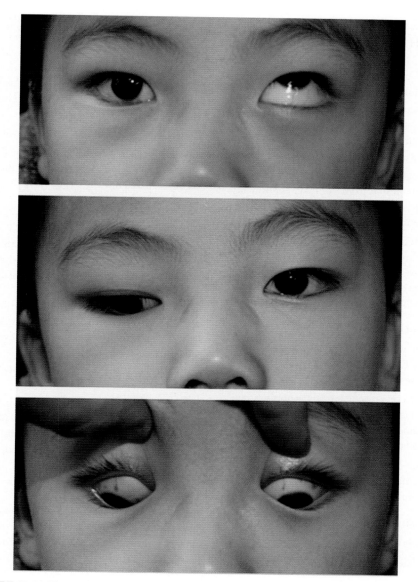

FIGURE 11-16. Monocular elevation deficiency. Monocular elevation deficiency of the right eye. Note the pseudoptosis of the right upper eyelid. (From Nelson LB, Olitsky SE. *A Color Handbook of Pediatric Clinical Ophthalmology*. London, England: Manson Publishing; 2011.)

CONGENITAL FIBROSIS OF THE EXTRAOCULAR MUSCLES

Epidemiology and Etiology

- CFEOM is a rare disease that occurs in approximately 1 in 230,000 people. Patients with CFEOM are usually born with ophthalmoplegia and ptosis (Fig. 11-17).

- Although the name of the syndrome suggests that it results from a primary abnormality of muscle, there is evidence that suggests that it may result from a primary abnormality of the cranial nerve's innervation of these muscles.

- There are four subtypes of CFEOM, and the genes have been localized for three of them. Both autosomal dominant and autosomal recessive inheritance patterns have been observed.

Signs and Symptoms

- When evaluating an individual with suspected CFEOM, a thorough family history should be obtained.

- CFEOM is present at birth, is nonprogressive, and is frequently associated with ptosis. Depending on the subtype, it may be unilateral or bilateral.

- The specific position of the eyes and pattern of movement define each clinical subtype of CFEOM.

Differential Diagnosis

- Double elevator palsy
- Third nerve palsy
- Chronic progressive ophthalmoplegia
- Thyroid-related strabismus

Diagnostic Evaluation

- A family history may reveal other relatives with a similar disorder. Genetic testing can confirm the diagnosis in some patients.

- Forced duction testing results are positive.

- During surgery, fibrotic bands can be found under the rectus muscles that must be located and severed to allow the eye to move during surgery.

Treatment

- The goal of surgical management in the general fibrosis syndrome is to center the eyes and improve the compensatory head posture. In patients with significant hypotropia, large recession or disinsertion of the inferior rectus muscles is indicated. However, elevation of the hypotropic eye accentuates the ptosis. Bilateral frontalis suspension is required soon after the strabismus surgery.

- Because these patients often do not have a Bell phenomenon, corneal drying may occur after ptosis surgery. Therefore, the eyelid should be elevated only to the upper pupillary border.

Prognosis

- These are very challenging patients and may require multiple surgeries to help reduce their compensatory head posture to provide comfortable vision.

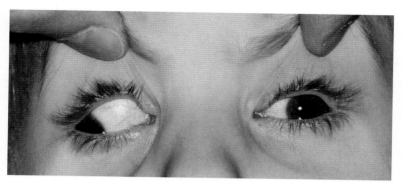

FIGURE 11-17. Congenital fibrosis of the extraocular muscles.

Index

Note: Page numbers followed by 'f' and 't' refer figures and tables respectively.